Yoga for All

Published by :
Lotus Press Publishers & Distributors

Yoga for All

Krishan Kumar Suman
M.A. B.T., Yogacharya, Ayurveda Ratna
Chief Editor: Yoga Manjari

Lotus PRESS

4735/22, Prakash Deep Building
Ansari Road, Darya Ganj,
New Delhi - 110002

Lotus Press : Publishers & Distributors
Unit No. 220, 2nd Floor, 4735/22, Prakash Deep Building,
Ansari Road, Darya Ganj, New Delhi- 110002
Ph.: 41325510, 98118-38000
• E-mail : lotuspress1984@gmail.com
www.lotuspress.co.in

Yoga for All

ISBN: 978-81-8382-235-0

Printed & Published by : **Lotus Press Publishers & Distributors**, New Delhi-02

Preface

There was a time when people did not fall ill due to simple life, pure food, pure environment, hard work and positive thinking. In this modern age we are facing many problems like pollution, crowd, adulteration in food stress and diseases. Only yogic lifestyle can save our miserable life.

According to 'Hatha Yoga Pradipika' ***Dynamic Health*** is explained like this—"a person enjoys good health, when he has slim body, joyous face, sonorous voice, sparking eyes, positive good health, virility, exuberance of vitality and possess radiance and a well timed nervous system. These are some of the characteristics of a 'Hatha Yogi'."

Dynamic health also means living a yogic life having a lot of strength and endurance, a sense of good feeling all the times, being *sattvic*, disciplined, smart, balanced, creative, broad minded, loving humanity and searching the ***Truth*** throughout one's long and happy life.

Yoga is therefore a way of life, a highly developed technique. It teaches us 'How to live rightly'? It ultimately leads an individual to self-realisation along with ***'Dynamic Health'***, complete unification with the pure consciousness of human existence. Yoga practice makes a man ***'Healthy in body as well as healthy in the mind.'***

Health is our birth right. To be healthy is natural and to fall sick is un-natural and sin. It is said, ***'Prevention is better than cure'***.

It must be borne in mind that health can't be had just by asking or wishing or by taking pills. Health can't be purchased. For remaining healthy one has to make a determined, persistent and consistent efforts, with self-imposed discipline.

Yoga is the only way to achieve the *'Dynamic Health'*. Yogic techniques were designed and perfected by the great *'Rishis'*. These techniques are most scientific, efficacious, easiest to learn and practice and has the stamp of thousands of years of experience by our great *'Rishis'*. Yoga is thus the only constructive and dynamic programme of 'Astanga yoga' is mainly the base of *'Dynamic Health'*.

There are so many books on yoga in the market but they represent for yogasana mostly. This book is totally different from them. It covers all the needful contents in details. Seventeen chapters have been included in it for deep study and practice of yoga.

'What is yoga' is cleared by several definitions. *'Why yoga*? is explained in thirteen points. *'A brief history of yoga'* is given alongwith the modern famous yoga centres. 'Yogic philosophy' is untouched in socalled books. Six schools of philosophy are explained in brief.

'All life is yoga' is discussed as yoga for better living. We should live in the world without any attachment, surrendering our every single work to the Divine. Only seven main streams of yoga have been explained in details.

'Yama and Niyama' are the fundamentals of *'Astanga yoga'*. Ten commandments (disciplinary guide lines) are discussed here in a simple way.

'Yogasana' the particular postures of the body, its importance, difference between simple exercises and yogasanas, directions about

yogasanas, Engligh names of yogasanas, classification of yogasanas, method and benefits of fifty one yogasanas are illustrated with diagrams. *'To avoid it'*—Some yogasanas should be avoided. Twelve practice programmes also given. Curative value of yogasanas is listed of forty eight diseases.

Before starting the yogasanas sixteen *exercises for flexibility* are illustrated with methods. Nineteen yogic mudras are explained for advance practice of yoga.

'Pranayama' (yogic breathing) is a very important part of yoga. Pran, Pranayama, its importance, its mechanism, instructions for pranayama, methods and exercises are given of some pranayamas.

'Pratyahara' 'Dharna' and *'Meditation'* are the advance Sadhana of yoga. Their meaning, importance, practice exercises, are explained in details. Seven chakras and methods of meditations are given. What is mind and how to control it? Is explained.

Without purification of body, mind and consciousness *'Dynamic Health'* can't be achieved. So many methods are given here. Yoga is a sure and successful means to control the sexual feelings. Yogic diet has a very important role in *'Dynamic Health'*. Food value and useful hints are given in the last chapter.

There are 134 figures in it to understand the theme easily. 16 pages are included of 39 coloured photos of some yogasanas, pranayamas and shuddhikriyas. This book is a good guide to every learner of yoga, ordinary type who wants to get *'Dynamic Health'* through yoga. Its language is simple. It is recommended that all the yogic techniques should be learnt from competent yogacharya or a trained yoga teacher.

I personally feel very much indebted to Mr. Uma Parshad Kaushal, a retired Vice Principal of government school, Delhi for going through the contents of the book and make corrections whenever necessary.

K.K. Suman

C-3/108C, Keshavpuram,

Delhi 110035

Contents

1

What is Yoga?

Yoga is very popular now-a-days and it is now well known to the whole world. It is not a mere exercise but yoga in real sense is union with God. All mystic practices and disciplines that lead to this Divine union are dealt under the word yoga.

Yoga is an evolution or a Science of consciousness. It is a perfect living style. It is the central part of Indian culture. All life is yoga and it is for all. Yoga is one of the very important six systems of the Indian philosophy. Yoga system is the 'grand father' of all the systems. These are methods of self-improvement at physical and mental level. It is based on deep love for God. It is an integrated system of techniques by which one develops ones hidden potentials to the fullest.

Yoga is an ancient Indian discipline of healing the body and mind through various asanas, breathing exercises, purification processes, *sattvic* diet and meditation. Yoga is a system of integral education not only of the body and the mind or the intellect, but also of the inner spirit. Yoga is a Science of life to develop the sixth sense to its fullness and to enjoy a blissful and peaceful life. It is essentially an art of understanding all about the soul.

Definition of Yoga

(1) "Yoga is a methodical effort towards self-perfection by the development of potentialities latent in the individual."

—*Sri Aurobindo*

Sri Aurobindo emphasises an all-round personality development –at the physical, mental, intellectual, emotional and spiritual levels.

(2) "Yogah Karmasu Kaushalam" —*Geeta*

योगः कर्मसु कौशलम्

Yoga is dexterity in action. The dexterity is bound to keep one ready for action in a relaxed attitude and efficiency is the outcome of all such actions.

(3) 'Yogah Chitta Vritti Nirodhah'

योगाश्चित्तवृत्ति निरोधः —*Patanjali*

Yoga is the inhibition of the modifications of the mind. This means that it prevents the contents of the mind from taking different forms. One can achieve control, suppression or inhibition of the activities and modifications of the mind (Chitta Vritties) by constant practice of yoga and non-attachment (अभ्यास एवं वैराग्य)।

(4) "Yoga may be defined as a process (journey) as well as a state or goal in many ways. Yoga is the science and art of quieting the subconscious mind a way of life, skill in action, union of thought word and deed, integration of our personality at all levels, the Science of conscious evolution and the method to attain as well as the state of emotional and mental equanimity."

—*Dr. A.B. Bhawanani*

What is not Yoga?

Yoga is not performing superhuman feats or acrobatics, as is sometimes falsely propagated by mass-media, especially in certain T.V. Programmes.

Yoga is not magic, miracle or a mystery. Yoga is not a religion. Yoga is not only a collection of physical exercises. It is something more comprehensive. Yoga is practised in two forms–internal and external (Antrang and Bahirang Yoga).

Why Yoga?

The world is full of chaos, because man has forgotten his 'self' and just exists at a lower animal stage of acquiring power and pelf for his own happiness.

1. Yoga helps to acquire a well-integrated personality at all levels—Physical, mental, emotional, intellectual and spiritual.
2. The first signs of entering yoga are lightness of body, health, thirstlessness of mind, clearness of complexion, a sweet voice, an agreeable fragrance and decantiness of excretions.
3. Yoga leads to *Sattvic Ahara* (Food), *Sattvic Vichara* (Positive thoughts), *Ideal Achara* (discipline) and *Vihara* (Healthy enjoyment).
4. Yoga develops awareness, willpower, good habits, peace, happiness and harmony etc. in life.
5. It gives us better understanding, self-confidence, higher abilities, a long life, security, love, sense of discrimination and intuition.
6. Yoga is the only gateway of a more elevated humanity, to a well-provided, progressive, war-free, harmonious and happy world.
7. It develops practice total ethical values in us by practice of Yama and Niyama.
8. It purifies our body through Shatkarmas.
9. Yoga develops maximum potential of senses through the practice of sense withdrawal, abstractions (Pratyahara).

10. Yoga removes the physical ailments. Its therapeutic aspect attracts the people.
11. Yoga provides smartness, good concentration, balance of mind, non-attachment, liberation, eternal bliss and perfection.
12. Yoga enhances our work efficiency, oneness with the world tension free life and cordial relationship.
13. Yoga purifies the mind by good deeds, *Swadhyaya* meditation and feeling of *vairagya.*

• • •

2

A Brief History of Yoga

Yoga has a lengthy history. Although the historical details are unclear, these writings are generally believed to data as far back as 6000 B.C. Archaeological evidence shows that yoga was practiced prior to 2000 B.C. by the inhabitants of the Indus Valley. Through the spoken words, the yogic tradition was passed on by teachers (Guru) to their pupils.

A major shift from oral to written tradition began by Aryans. After 2000 B.C. The Aryans developed the Deowani—Sanskrit language, which later took hold as the canonical language of the Hindu Scriptures. Vedas, Upnishads, Brahman granthas, Smarities, Aranyakas were all written in Sanskrit, and because the forerunners of yoga are found in these works, Sanskrit became the accepted standard for yogic vocabulary.

Scattered elements of the yogic tradition were evident throughout the Hindu scriptures, but yoga had yet to evolve into an independent school of thought. It was not until 300 B.C. that yoga, as an organised grouping of principles and practices, began to take form. About this time, a number of Philosophical systems emerged from the basic Upanishadic teachings. Each systems outlined a path to spiritual salvation. Yoga gained immense popularity for its practical approach to spiritual concerns; bringing spiritual liberation through a series of physical and mental exercise.

The person most responsible for systematising yoga was the Indian Philosopher Patanjali. Sometime around 200 B.C. Patanjali bolstered the move from oral to written tradition. In the classical treatise yoga sutras. Patanjali codified in writing a large body of yogic precepts and processes. But Patanjali was not the creator of a new and revolutionary mode of thought. He merely gave orderly expression to pre-existing yogic doctrine.

According to Maharishi *Yagyavalkya* Hiranyagarbha Rishi was the first preacher of yoga. Some believe that Lord Shiva is the founder of Yoga. According to the Gita Lord Krishna tells to Arjuna that *Bhagwan* himself told to the king Vivaswana (Manu) and king Manu told to king Ekswaku. Like this, many Raja rishis learned the yoga. Sometime after '*Dwapar*' this yoga disappeared.

Maharishi Kashyapa, Kapil, Aditi Manu, Dadhichi revived yoga. Many streams came in the light. Now-a-days some famous yogis are working for yoga and they brought it to the ground level making it available to every one. More than two thousand books are written on yoga. Some magazines (Yoga, Yog Manjari, Yoga Vidhya, Yoga Varsha, Yoga Sundesh etc.) are spreading the message of yoga-culture. Media is also helping a lot in this field.

Now-a-days the leading yogic centres working in this field are: *Shivanada* Ashram. Rishikesh, Swami Satyananda Saraswati Ashram of Ganga Darshan Munger, Bihar, Vivekananda Kendra Yoga Research Foundation, Mangalore. Kuvalayanandashram, Pune, Maharashtra, Bharatiya Yoga Sansthan, (Rohini, Delhi), Maharishi Mahesh Yogi's Ashram Noida (U.P.), Swami Ram Dev, Haridwar, Uttarakhand, Maharishi Bharthari, Chennai, Tamilnadu, Ma

Nirmala Devi for Kurdalini Shakti (Sahaja Yoga). Sri Aurobindo Ashram Puducherry. Param Hansa Yogananda Ashram, Ranchi (Jharkhand), Swami Jyotirmayananda Ashram, Lal Bagh, Loni (Near Delhi), Swami Gitananda Ashram, Puducherry, Kailash Ashram Rishikesh (U.P.), Delhi Yoga Sabha, Bhama Shah Marg, New Delhi and Yoga Vigyan Sansthan Ashok Vihar, Delhi.

• • •

3
Yogic Philosophy

Yogic Philosophy is one of the world's greatest philosophy. It is profound, penetrating, enlightening and enduring. And yogic practices constitute some of the world's greatest religious endeavours. Whether pursued in conjunction with the metaphysics of Patanjali or with other metaphysical outlooks, yogic practices embody some ideas, ideals and feelings which are common to all religions. Yoga works because it embodies certain psychological principles which are true for all times and ages and all sects of human life.

Yoga philosophy is essentially humanistic. As much as any philosophy, Like Samkhya philosophy, it is neither theistic nor atheistic. Yoga is one of the six systems of Indian philosophy (Darshanas). 'Darshana' means 'View Point' or 'Vision' from the root 'drs' to see; 'to comprehend'; 'to contemplate'.

The six schools of philosophy developed in the post–upnishadic period. For the theory behind its practice, yoga borrows extensively from the Samkhya system, and the two names are often linked with a hyphen. The remaining four philosophies also paired, giving Samkhya-yoga, Mimansa-vedanta, and Nyaya-vaisesika. Yoga has become popular as it is not only a philosophy of life but is of immense value with its practical aspects is human life.

Samkhya Yoga

There is an old Indian saying, "There is no knowledge equal to the Samkhya, and no power equal to the yoga". Samkhya yoga is mainly a natural philosophy. The leading Samkhya source text is Kapila's '**Samkhya Sutras**' and the key work in the philosophy and practice of the yoga of meditation is Patanjali's 'Yoga Sutras' are condensed statements—the word is usually translated as '**aphorism**'.

Samkhya's approach to liberations by way of metaphysical knowledge, intellectually accepted, where as yogi's approach is by way of psycho-physiological techniques and controls, though it uses Kapila's account of evolution, consciousness, the body-mind problem, and so on, as a theoretical support.

Kapila explained eternal evolution and dissolution in the universe in terms of ***Purusha*** (Soul/Spirit) and ***Prakriti*** (basic substance/Body), and the later's evolutes. But yoga, taking Samkhya's philosophy, added a Supreme Being, a liberated ***Purush***. Thus, God appears in Patanjali's Sutras, without fitting easily into the philosophical and metaphysical teaching of that work.

Vedanta Yoga

'Veda' means knowledge, 'Anta' means last. Samkhya yoga holds to the doctrine of the purality of souls (Purushas) with Ishvara (God) as a special Purusha. The best known branch of vedanta philosophy is ***Advaita Vedanta***, founded by Adi Shankŕacharya, whose central tenet is non-duality. Soul, Atman and Purusha are the same. God or Brahaman are the same. ***Purusha*** is pure consciousness (Chitta), eternal spaceless, passive, the seer/witness.

It is the unchanging clear light against which the mind thoughts and images becomes visible not the images on the mental screen, but the projectors illumination. Buddhi reflects the ***Purusha.***

Prakriti, the basic substance of the universe serves ***Purusha.*** Purusha initiates-cosmic evolution by coming into proximity with matter.

Prakriti

The basic substance of things (Prakriti/body) can be divided into three inherent qualities called *Gunas*. These are *tamas, rajas* and *sattva*—or inertia, energy, and intelligence respectively. Alternative definitions of *sattva* are 'orderliness', 'purity', and 'illumination'. These three qualities or *Gunas* combine to make up all the objects of Nature. The predominance of a *guna* in a thing determined its essential nature.

Tamas represents mass, resistance, stability, solidity, and durability,. *Rajas* is the kinetic principle, responsible for the activity within the atom, and for change and motion everywhere in Nature, within the mind it is responsible for the coming and going of thoughts and flow of the emotions *Sattva* that makes for orderliness, *sattva* is found in its most characteristic elements in the working of consciousness. It represents a pure and light quality.

There are five tanmatras into the five gross atoms—earth, water, fire, air and ether. These make up 24 categories, with soul they become 25 in total.

Tattva's 25 Categories

1. Purusha (Soul)
2. Prakriti, Basic Substance
3. Mahat, Buddhi, Cosmic consciousness
4. Ahankara 'I'-sense

The Six Senses

5. Sight
6. Hearing
7. Smell
8. Taste
9. Touch
10. Manas (mind as coordinating faculty)

The Five Motor Organs

11. Hands
12. Feet
13. Speech organs
14. Excretory organs
15. Generative organs

The Five Potentials (Tanmatras)

16. Light
17. Sound
18. Smell
19. Taste
20. Touch

The Five Atoms

21. Earth
22. Water
23. Fire
24. Air
25. Ether

States of Consciousness

1. Waking
2. Dream
3. Deep Sleep
4. Turya

States of Jiva in the three states of Jiva

1. Self
2. Ignorance
3. Ego
4. Mind
5. Senses
6. Objects

Seven States of Wisdom

1. Shubechha (Good Aspiration)
2. Vicharana (Reflection)
3. Tanumanasi (Subtlety of Mind)
4. Sattwapatti (Pervasion of Purity)
5. Asamsakti (Detachment)

6. Padarthabhavana (Absence of World)
7. Turya (Transcendence)

Man's Objectives (Purushartha)

1. Dharma
2. Artha
3. Kama
4. Moksha

Four Principles of Life

1. Vairagya (Non-attachment)
2. Vivek (Understanding)
3. Shuddhta (Purity)
4. Moksha (Will of Completeness), (Liberation from Bondages)

Four States of Life

1. Brahamacharyashrama upto 25 years for studying and learning.
2. Grahasthashrama, 25-50 years for family life.
3. Vanprasthashrama, 50-75 years for social service.
4. Sanyasashrama, 75-100 years for feeling of detachment and gradual withdrawal, self-realisation.

Aadi, Acharya

1. Hiranyagarsha
2. Patanjali

Yoga Darshana by Patanjali

Four Chapters of Yoga Darshan

There are 4 Pada and 195 Sutras in Yogadarshana.

1. Samadhi Pada 51
2. Sadhana Pada 55
3. Vibhooti Pada 55
4. Kaivalya Pada 34

1. **Samadhi Pada:** It is an explanation of 3 sutras (2, 3, 4) how to control the mind, it is described by concentration and Sampragyata Samadhi (Trance). There are four parts of this kind trance-vitarka, vichara, Ananda and Asmita.

2. **Sadhana Pada:** In this chapter five obstacles (kleshas) are described such as—Avidhya (ignorance), Asmita (egoism), Raga (desire), Dwesha (hate/aversion), Abhinivesha (greed/possessiveness). These are the source of sorrow.

   Astanga yoga has 8 limbs—Yama, Niyama, Asana Pranayama, Pratyahara, Dharana, Dhyana and Samadhi. All these have been described in details in this book.

3. **Vibhuti Pada:** Dharana and Samadhi are called Sanyama. In this pada states of supper consciousness has been explained.

4. **Kaivalya Pada:** In this pada the doubts about the chitta (mind) and its states and solution are described, 'who am I'? the riddle is disclosed. What is kaivalya is explained.

   Body is the embodiment of the universe. Our body is the cover of our individual soul. Abound soul may suffer reincarnation many times because it remains attached to a subtle body whose karmic effects require other lives in which work out its fate. But once a soul has been liberated from body completely, it is freed from further incarnation.

• • •

4

Yoga for Better Living

Yoga is a way of life. Sri Aurobindo says, "All life is yoga". It means our every action should be on yogic pattern. Yoga is a process of evolution of the self physically, mentally, morally, intellectually, emotionally, socially and spiritually. Yoga is a path of all round development. Our every moment should be full of happiness, harmonious, dedicated, tension free and for Divine.

Sri Aurobindo suggests to live a yogic life-one should adopt this formula of Sadhana and better living—*aspiration, rejection* of obstacles, bad habits and negative thoughts; the third is *surrender* to Divine. Ultimately we should live being a karmayogi.

Astanga yoga, geeta yoga, upnisadas guidelines and our old yogic literature inspire us how to live in this world. Yoga teaches us a wonderful discipline through Yama and Nyama.

Five universal commandments (Yamas) aimed at creating better life and better world; not harming anyone or anything, truthfulness, non-stealing, leading a godly and chaste life and being non-grasping.

Five personal disciplines (Niyama); cleanliness, contentedness, self-discipline, self-study and study of scriptures, and dedication to God.

Due to practice of postures, Pranayama, mudras shat karmas we get sound health and remove the ailments because body is the base of all activities.

Detachment from worldly activities, developing a non-attached attitude of body and mind. Meditation and trance lead towards our goal of happiness, health and realisation or service to the humanity.

"Yoga is an art of opening the unconscious part of our being" along with we learn the art of living in favourable and unfavourable situations, conflicts, tension, ego problems and human relations. How to control our mind and senses? How to transform our Chittavritis? how to remove the kleshas, how to purify our Antahkarana?

Yoga teaches us the effect of *tamsic*, *rajsic* and *sattvic* diet. We become what we eat. Sattvic food is recommended by yoga. One should eat with awareness, good feeling and a calmly mind.

Yoga develops personality at physical, mental, emotional, intellectual and spiritual levels, Yoga gives the chance to get relaxed muscles, strong but flexible body parts, active systems. It gives us the power of imagination, creativity and steadfastness will power. Calming down the mind and balancing the mind, technique of facing the challenges of life, polite behaviour, positive attitude. Concentration and detachment, spiritual development effects the whole society in peace and harmony, inner divinity in man are all aspects of life.

There are mainly four streams of yoga—Karma yoga, Bhakti yoga, Raja yoga and Gyana yoga. Yoga develops the thinking of 'Work is worship'. Controlling of emotions, better understanding, psychic control respectively. So that our life becomes joyful with the help of 'Abhyasa' and 'Vairagya'.

The yoga of life is a continuous meditation, where each thought, word and action is done with full awareness and in a state of relaxation. Yoga treats the person at his fundamental root cause. There are no specifics. It offers an education in living at 4 levels. ***Ahara*** (Food) ***Achara*** certain practices and routines followed in a disciplined way, ***Vichara*** correct type of thing and thought patterns and disciplined emotional balance. ***Vihara*** correct plan of recreation and rejuvenation. Thus Ahara, Achara, Vichara and Vihara fit into the total concept of better living where a balance is struck between one's work, recreation, food and habits of thought to make the wheels life run harmoniously.

Yoga is interested in to create deeper awareness of our action, thoughts, behaviour, health, peace and understanding ourselves, our duties to ourselves and society. Yoga inspires for 'simple living and high thinking', 'early to bed early to rise', getting harmony of the body, mind and soul to live for Divine.

We should follow the guidelines of Geeta—The essence of Sri Madbhagavad Geeta is given here.

- Why are you unnecessarily worring? Whom do you fear? Who can kill you? Soul is not born, nor does it die.
- What has happened for the best. What is happening is happening for the best. Don't brood over the past. Don't worry about the future. The present is on. Give the importance to the present movement with full awareness.
- What have you lost, that you are weeping? What have you brought, that you have lost? What have you made, that has been destroyed? You brought not anything. What you have, you got from here. What was given here. What you took, you took from this universe. What you gave, you gave unto this universe. You have come empty handed and shall go empty handed. What is yours today was somebody else's in the past and will be somebody else's in the future. You think

it is yours and are deeply engrossed in it. This attachment is the cause of all your sorrow.

- 'Change is the Law of Life' What you call Death is life itself. In a moment you are a millionaire in the very next moment you are a poor man. Mine-yours; Small-Big; Ours-theirs; Remove this from your mind, then everything is yours and you are everybody's.
- This body is not yours, nor you are of this body. Earth, Air, Fire, Water and Ether comprise this body and unto this shall it turn. But the soul is Immortal, then what are you?
- Surrender unto the Lord. He is the Ultimate Support. He who experiences this is completely free from Fear, Worry and Despair.
- Whatever you do, other it unto Him. By this you shall forever experience Eternal bliss". (Lord Shrikrishna)

• • •

5

Main Streams of Yoga

There are four to seven famous streams. Swami Vivekananda puts four streams as work, worship, philosophy and psychic control. Laya yoga and Hatha yoga are famous branches of yoga. Let us discuss them briefly.

(A) Karm Yoga

Karm yoga is a selfless service without attachment, without ego, done as a duty, surrendered to the Divine and according to the law of Karma. Karma yoga is called 'the yoga of Action' but it must be understood that a special quality of action is intended, this special quality at its purest is called actionless action (Niskam Karma), and results from non-attachment (Vairagya). In the Bhagwad Gita, in which the most inspired instruction in 'the way of action' is to be found, the need for non-attachment is stressed again and again, but this is only really complete when the individual has found and lives in his self, which is untouched by action and is over and about it as pure being.

Karm yoga is wisdom in work and action. The Karm yogi's actions are marked by pose of body, mind and spirit. Each action, when performed with right intention becomes contemplative.

In Karm yoga, Love and duty have become one, duties become sources of happiness. Karm yoga means service and work without clinging to the fruits of action. One should perform the ***Sattvic Karm*** in his daily life for others of unto God. In Gita ***'Yogah Karmsu Kaushlam'*** and ***'Samatvam yoga Uchayate'*** are preferred for Karm yoga. Lord Krishna taught the lesson of Karm yoga to Arjuna. This is explained in Gita in details.

With Karm yoga we can purify our Antahkaran. We become unselfish, egoless, lover of humanity, instrument of God, happy and we are able to realise our reality which is the centre of unlimited bliss.

(B) Bhakti Yoga

The control of emotions is the key to the path of Bhakti yoga (Worship). It teaches Divine love and devotion through emotional control and ethical conduct. Bhakti or Devotion is Supreme Love directed towards God. There are two kinds of Bhakti; Kamya and Niskamya. There are two kinds of Niskamya Bhakti—

(1) Vaidhi or external puja and japa etc.

(2) Ragatmika or Prema (internal)

There are nine modes of Bhakti—Sharvan, Kirtan, Sumiran, Padsevan, Archana, Vandana, Dasya, Sakhya and Atma-Nivedan.

The seeker as Uddhava tells two kinds of Bhakti.

(3) *Artharthi*—He who has the desire obtain some object. Dhurva is an example

(4) *Gyani*—The wise as Shukadeva etc.

For God realisation there are Nine Modes of Bhakti—

1. Shravan (Hearing)

Listening to the glories of the Lord. Raja Prikshit is the example for this. He knew he was going to die in a week but got so absorbed in hearing the glories of the Lord that even fear of death was overcome.

2. Kirtan (Chanting)

This helps a person in mastering the ego. The main examples are the Mira Bai and Chaitanya Maha Prabhu. They merged themselves in singing the glories of the Lord Krishna.

3. Sumiran (Remembering)

To remember God with every breath of life. Dhurva is the ideal example for this. He prayed to get the Kingdom of his father. Pleased with him the Lord appeared and asked, "What do you want?" He forget all as he was so much in bliss he wanted Bhakti and Bhakti alone and nothing else.

4. Padsevan (Adortion of the Lotus Feet)

Real service can only of the Lord by a pure heart and this heart can be cleansed with the dust of the Guru's lotus feet only. The very first mahamantra that Bhagwan gave was.

मनस भज रे गुरु चरणम्
दुस्तर भव सागर तरणम्।

(O man! worship the Lotus feet of the Guru. Difficult it is to cross over this ocean of life.)

When we bow down—this, directly or indirectly brings humility, the only friend and throws out the devils of pride.

5. Archana (Offerings)

All the prayers and worship to be done with the proper rituals. Raja Ambrish is the ideal example for this type. Once he requested Rishi Durvasa to have a meal at his place but in a moment of anger Durvasa was about to curse him when Lord Vishnus Sudarshan Chakra attacked the Rishi but none could help him. Ultimately the Rishi saved his life by taking shelter with the King Ambrish whom he wanted to curse. This is the power of Archana, oneness of Bhagwan and Bhakta.

6. Vandana (Adoration)

To see Him everywhere Bhakta Akrura is the best example for this type. When he went to Braja (Vrindavan)—where he saw the signs of Divine feet of the Lord—Kissed the place—Saw him in every particle.

7. Dasya (Servitude)

Thou are the Master and I am Thy humble Servant. This is the dominant feeling. Hanumana is the ideal example for this. He told Lord Rama when he asked to Hanumana, "Who am I".

8. Sakhya (Fellow-mate)

The cowherd boys and Arjuna are the ideal examples. This Bhakti is the most informal-no secrets bring oneness. Krishna washed Sudama's feet with his own hands and drank that very water. That is the intimacy that is the oneness.

9. Atma-Nivedan (Self-Surrender)

Raja Bali and Prahlad are the ideal examples for this. They dedicated all the actions to him with a feeling of complete surrender.

Some Rishis have named a few more types of Bhakti, as—Shant Bhava (Peaceful), Vatsalya (Parental Love), and Madhurya (Love of a wife for a husband) etc.

Due to Bhakti yoga the Bhakta, the devotee gets peace, happiness. Confidence, simplicity, deep faith in religion. He develops love towards all human beings etc.

(C) Gyan Yoga

Gyan Yoga is the method of realisation through constant investigation about the real nature of self, ego and the universe. This path of philosophy is apt for the keen intellectuals and is centred around the analysis of 'Happiness', the vital contribution of Upnishads. Also, many other fundamental questions regarding mind, the world outside and inside and reality are taken up.

This path of knowledge is the process of reasoning that uncovers the deep-seated truths underlying life. Renunciation of the unreal brings a better understanding of the true meaning of life. The Gyan yogi is a philosopher who wishes to go beyond the visible. The search for the ultimate reality is not complete until the Divine origin of human kind is discovered and accepted.

A student in the path of Gyan Yoga develops the four means of salvation, viz., Vivek, Vairagya, Sad-Sampatti (Shama, Dama, Titiksha, Uparati, Sradha, Samadhana) and Mumkshutwa. Then he hears the Srutis (Sravan). Then he does Manan (reflection) and Nididhyasan (constant meditation). He meditates on the right significance of Om and the great Mahavakya—TAT TWAM ASI, which can note the identity of Jiva and Paramatma. This is Antaranga Sadhna. Then he gets Atma Sakshatkara or self-realisation.

(D) Hatha Yoga

This system, aims to achieve the union by bringing, the body to its highest state of development and under the complete control of the mind. According to Swatmarama an old authority, on this yoga, declares in the 'Hathayoga-Pradipika' that Hathayoga is the staircase which leads to the goal of Rajayoga.

The term Hatha originates from two Sanskrit root sounds '**Ha**' and '**Tha**'. The sound Ha represents the solar flow in Pingla channel and Tha represents the lunar flow in Ida channel. Hatha yoga is to bring perfect harmony between the flows of Pingla (Positive and hot) and Ida (negative and cool). The term Hatha yoga used in this context means the regulation of breath or union of the two breaths into one.

Traditionally, the system of Hatha yoga consists mainly in the following disciplines:

1. Asanas (Physical Postures)

2. Pranayamas (Breath Control)
3. Mudras (Body Gestures)
4. Bandhas (Energy Locks)
5. Satkarmas (Six Purifying Techniques)

A Hath yogi is interested in awakening the Kundalini Shakti that is lying dormant in the basa of Muladhara chakra. Yogi enters into Nirvikalpa Samadhi and attains mukti as well as Bhakti (spiritual enjoyment). He experiences four awasthas while practising pranayama the Arambha Awastha, the Ghata Awastha, the Parichaya Awastha and the Nispatti Awastha.

Hatha Yoga is practised by majority of people for its practical benefits to the health of the glands, vital organs and nervous system. Japa and meditation are included in its Sadhana.

(E) Gita Yoga

Introduction

Sri Madbhagwad Gita is a tremendous holy book of yoga. Its meaning is '**Song of the Divine**'. It was written some 5000 years ago by Rishi Vyas. It is a part of famous epic 'Mahabharata'. It is given the status of 'Shruti' and 'Pancham Veda' as it contains the essence of the upnishadic teachings of vedas. The central theme of the Bhagwat Gita is Sanyasa i.e., renunciation. It means exploration of the purpose of human life. It states that renunciation is a desired goal.

Gita is respected and honoured by all religions. It is practical yoga. Its theme is given in short but complete. Wideness is seen in its words. It touches all the aspects of life such as—meditation, concentration, japa, tapa, love, faith, bhakti (devotion), Karma, behaviour, more than hundred 'Bhasyas' (explanation) are written on it. The great persons followed its teachings. It is an inspiring guide.

There are 18 chapters, 18 yogas are implemented in it such as—1. Visad yoga, 2. Samkhya yoga, 3. Karm yoga, 4. Yoga of wisdom, 5. Yoga of renunciation of action, 6. Yoga of meditation, 7. Gyan yoga, 8. Akshar brahm yoga, 9. Guhya yoga, 10. Vibhuti yoga, 11. Viswa roop darshan yoga, 12. Bhakti yoga, 13. Yoga of distinction, 14. Guna-traya vibhaga yoga, 15. Purshottama yoga, 16. Devasur sampada yoga, 17. Shradha trya yoga, 18. Moksha sanyasa yoga.

There are about 700 verses (slokas) in it. It is written in Sanskrit language. Lord Krishna gave the knowledge of Truth to Arjuna to implement his duty. Gita is a way of life, research of life and art of man-making. Gita is a scheme of life. It is a glory of self-restraint. Some say she is a mother who leads for a better life and yogic life.

Gita Teaches

Gita teaches us efficiency of Karma, Karm yoga, Samatva buddhi, Sthith pragya state, soul is immortal, trigunas, to live like a lotus. There is no difference between man to man at soul level. We should try to purify the chitta. We should develop sattvic nature. One can achieve the essence of yoga through practice and non-attachment. Om is the mantra which provides 'Parampad' (God realisation/Atma Sakshatkara). Be satisfied in the soul. Learn to give not to take. Do selfless service. Perform meditation regularly. See God in every creature. Do your duty sincerely. Control the obstacle of mind. See the life as a witness.

Lord Krishna says, "Leave all things behind and come to me for thy salvation. I will make thee free from the bondage of sins. Fear no more". (18/67)

"Set thy heart upon thy work, but never on its fruit. Work not for the reward, but never cease to do your work." (2/47).

In Gita we find that the work can be pure and noble. That is why Sri Krishna says, "offer to me all your work and let your mind rest on the Supreme. Be free from vain hopes and selfish thoughts and with inner peace, fight your fight" (3/30).

Gita inspires all to live like a yaga. Think for other do for others. Gita does not inspire not to work but to do some work without any selfish motto without attachment feelings and ego. It teaches us to control the mind and how to live in this world.

(F) Swara Yoga

The Science of Swara Yoga is an ancient one and has been gifted to the humanity by the Indian saints and *munis* for leading a healthy and prosperous life, longevity and to achieve the goal of liberation.

Normally a person does not breathe a evenly through both the nostrils, but alternately. The breath in a human being alternates cyclically from one nostril to another, approximately after 60 to 120 minutes the breath flows right, left and both the nostrils they are named as

1. Surya Swara—Right Swara, Pingla nadi (Hot)
2. Chandra Swara—Left Swara, Ida nadi (Cold)
3. Susumna Swara—The Saraswati air flows from the both nostrils

In a swara five elements (Tatvas) flow for some minutes as Jal, Prithivi, Vayu, Agani and Akash respectively. There are 72000 nadis in the whole body but Ida, Pingla and Susumna are the main nadis. They work scientifically and automatically with a natural timetable.

The word 'Hatha' in Hathayoga is composed of two words. 'Ha' and 'Tha' 'Ha' stands for Pingla Nadi and Tha for Ida Nadi. Here the word 'Nadi' means the pathway for flow of pranic energy (Bioenergy) with the combination of Ida and Pingla. The pranic energy flows through Susumna (right and left nostrils). This stage is for meditation or Samadhi. Ida Nadi lies on the left side and the

Pingla Nadi on right side of spinal column and Susumna Nadi in the spinal column.

The good, permanent deeds are done in Ida (Chandra Swara). Activities laborious work and temporary deeds are done in Pingla (right swara). There are the lists of their jobs done in their duration

(1) Puraka Sakasar Shwas

Rechaka Hakaar Prashwas

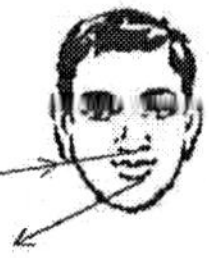

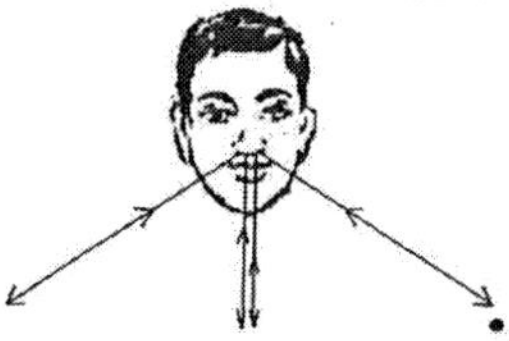

(2)

- **Pingla (Hot)**
- Surya Swara
- HA
- Odd
- Rajoguni
- Obstacle For gents

- Susumna
- Mixed
- Pranic energy
- For meditation
- Bad result of work
- Satoguni

- **Ida (Cold)**
- Chandra Swara
- Tha
- Even
- Tamo guni success
- For ladies

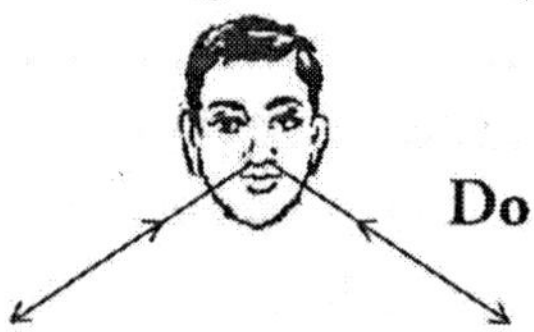

Do These Jobs in Pingla

(3)

- **Hard Work**
- Temporary work
- Food
- Natural call
- Bath, Sharing
- Cold things to eat/drink

- **Light Work**
- Permanent Work
- Drink water
- Natural call of urine
- Hot things to eat
- Donation

- Sleeping
- Coming home
- Sale
- Exercise
- Written Work
- Loan
- Shat Karmas
- Mountaineering
- Attraction etc.

- Flow should be more lengthy in day time
- Journey
- Medicine
- Friendship
- Business
- Opening
- Education Starting
- Deeksha
- Marriage
- Building the home
- Good work etc.

(4)

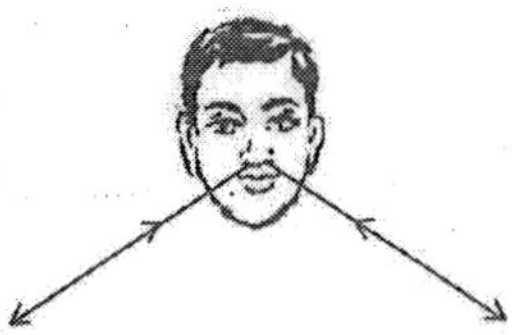

- Working Swara
- Living
- Fruitful
- Use this side first
- Positive Result
- Have Friends this sides

- Not Working Swara
- Dead Swara
- Fruitless Result
- Negative Result
- Keep this side who are against you.

(5) Tattva

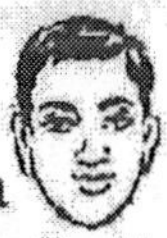

Tattva	Distance	Duration
1. Akash (Space)	0 Angul flow	4 minutes
2. Vayu (Air)	8 Angul flow	8 minutes
3. Agani (Fire)	4 Angul flow	12 minutes
4. Jal (Water)	16 Angul flow	16 minutes
5. Prithvi (Earth)	12 Angul flow	20 minutes
		1 Hour

Natural Breathing Flow

Krishn Paksha (Dark Fortnight)		Shukla Paksha (Bright Fortnight)	
Day Starts	Tithis	Tithis	
First from Right Nostril Surya	1, 2, 3	1, 2, 3	Day Starts from ← left Swara
Day Starts First from Left Nostril Moon Swara	4, 5, 6	4, 5, 6	Day Starts from ←right Swara
Day Starts First from Sun Swara	7, 8, 9	4, 5, 6	Day Starts from ←left Swara
Day Starts First from Moon Swara	10, 11, 12	4, 5, 6	Day Starts from ←right Swara
Day Starts First from Sun Swara	13, 14, 30	4, 5, 6	Day Starts from ←left Swara

Day starts according to this time table. It is the natural time table. 60 minutes flows from one nostril. The next swara if changed automatically. If there is any change in this said time table. It must be changed according to this time table otherwise there will be mental disturbances, loss of money, bed news, loss of dear things, death and disease may be. This time table is counted since sunrising to sun set.

Wrong Swara

Normally, one nostril flows for one hour alternatively. If **left Swara** (Chandra Swara/Ida Nadi) runs continuous by from sun rising the result will be like this—

4 hours continuous give	• rheumatic pain
4 hours 48 minutes	• Trouble from enemy
One day	• Mental disturbance

2nd day	• Loss of money
3rd day	• Journey
4th day	• Loss of position
5th day	• Struggle and trouble
10th day	• Misfortune
15th day	• Trouble
30th day	• Unauspicious, misfortune
45th day	• Possibility of death

- If in bright forth nights, it flows from right instead of left from the sunrise some tragedy may occur. If it flows from middle (susumna) on the first day of each month then there is no loss or gain.
- If susumna runs for two days, half-half pahar (+pahar = 3 hours) foreign tour and good luck is indicated.
- If it runs continuously from right in the night and left in the day, the day, long life is possible.
- If breathing flows for 4 hours at a time from either nostril the physical weakness is felt.
- When right breath runs for:
  - — 1.36 mts. stomach disorder/loss of money
  - — 4.38 mts. financial difficulty
  - — 5.08 mts. disease
  - — 8.24 mts. betrayal from friends
  - — 24.00 Serious illness related heat.
- If wrong Swara (Left/right) flows i.e., left instead of right or right instead of left flows for:

— First 3 hours gets	Worry
— Next 3 hours gets	Loss of money
— For 15 hours	Loss in position
— For 18 hours	Failure
— For 21-24 hours	Trouble

Change of Swara

- The trouble can be reduced by changing the swara according to the schedule.
  1. Stand on right foot for sometime, left swara will start soon.
  2. Press the opposite jaw which side you want to flow the air. Suppose you want to flow the right swara press the left jaw.
  3. Lie on the opposite side of the flowing nostril or press the side with a pillow.
  4. Inhale from the running nostril and exhale forcefully from the other side. Repeat this process.
  5. Stop the active nostril by fingers/plugging a cotton or cloth ball.
  6. Brisk walking, running and exercise also can change the swara.

Important Rules in Daily Life

- In Susumna the Worldly deeds are prohibited. Some important rules of swara yoga of general interest:

1. One should start taking major meals of the day in Solar Swara (Right Nostril)
2. One should attend natural call of latrine in Solar (Surya) Swara for easy defection and managing constipation.
3. One should attend the natural call of urine in lunar (Chandra) Swara for restricting the useful ingredients of blood from excretion.
4. One should go for bath and also for shaving activities in Solar Swara.
5. One should take article of hot potency like ginger, garlic, coffee, tea etc., and also the articles of liquid nature in Lunar Swara (Left Nostril)
6. One should intake the article of cold potency like curd, milk, radish, ice cream etc., in Surya Swara.

7. One should go for sleep in Solar Swara at night.
8. In case of having bath in Chandra Swara, you might be catch cold.
9. Intake of cold potency article in Chandra Swara may cause cold or rheumatism etc.
10. One should not have betel chewing in Surya Swara to avoid bileousness, urinary disorders etc.
11. One should have defect the flow of swara at the time of a particular trouble/disease in the body like headache, common cold, hypertension, gastric, acidity, asthmatic attack etc., and try to have flow of other swara artificially by changing the side, he will be surely relieved of the trouble after flow of other swara within 30-60 minutes.
12. One should perform the act of donation in the inhaling phase of Chandra Swara.
13. The intake of pure honey helps in flow of Surya Swara as a stimulation as well as for its durability.
14. The intake of pure ghee helps stimulation as well as durability of Chandra Swara.
15. In case of poisoning of right nature the flow of Chandra Swara provides assistance for counteraction.
16. The practice of Nadishodhan pranayama (80 times a day) helps in changing of Swara at one's own will.
17. Flow of Chandra Swara in the day time will help in the management of Hypertension and Surya Swara at night in low blood pressure.
18. The intake of medicine during Surya Swara for the disease caused by cold and in Chandra Swara for disease caused by heat will help in early recovery. Indulgence in sex during flow of same swara of the two partners will not cause pregnancy and this fact might be helpful in family planning.

(G) Astanga Yoga (Raja Yoga)

Raja yoga is the method of realising the God or Kaivalya through mental mastery. Raja yoga (Psychic control) gives a practical and easy approach to reach higher states of consciousness. It is based on the Antarang yoga of Patanjali Astanga yoga system. This is the most systematic method for attaining the highest state of meditation. It is the yoga of wisdom, control, harmony and equanimity, which embraces the accumulation of knowledge, esoteric, experience, arousing of psychic powers, philosophy and meditation. Raja yoga was propounded by Maharishi Patanjali. It is eight fold system. These limbs are listed below in order:

1. **Yamas (Abstinences) The disciplines:** Restrains of desires-social behaviour not to harm others. These are five,
   1. Ahimsa (Non-violence)
   2. Satya (Truthfulness)
   3. Asteya (Non-Stealing)
   4. Brahmacharya (Continence)
   5. Aprigraha (Non-Avariciousness)
2. **Niyamas (observances) personal character:** For improvement of oneself.
   1. Shouch—outer and inner cleanliness
   2. Santosh—Contentment
   3. Tap—Purificatory Action
   4. Swadhyaya—Self-study and study of scriptures.
   5. Ishwar Pranidhan—Dedication of all actions to God.

   The Yama and Niyama are interdependent. These are like two feet necessary for ascending the ladder of eight limbs of yoga. These are foundation stones for next 6 steps of the ladder. Without good character or moral practice of niyamas leads to downfall. Perfection of yamas is called Siddhi.

3. **Asanas (Postures) control of Body:** Yogasanas are the best and are Scientific exercises. Yogasanas give health and vitality necessary for yoga. Practice of yogasanas make you feel the 'Joy of living' in every nerve and fibre of your being. Yogasanas tone up the muscles and repair the tissues. Yogasanas are beneficial for meditation, good health and to remove the diseases. The Asanas should be steady and easy according to Patanjali.

   Yogasanas cultivate precision of movement and mental ability, helping you into purifying the body. They also increase flexibility. They are very helpful to every body.
4. **Pranayama (Breath Control):** The vital force known as Prana gives motion to all the organs of the body. Pranayamas are more useful than Asanas. The main benefits of Pranayamas are given below:

   Development of seminal energy, longevity, healthy body-systems, preparation of meditation, mental powers, purification of the body and mind. Purification of chitta and awakening of kundalini shakti etc. There are about 50 types of pranayamas.
5. **Pratyahara (Abstraction/Sense Withdrawal):** Detachment of the senses from their objects of enjoyment is called Pratyahara. Pratyahara is the initial process of turning the attention inwards of inhibiting the reception of the bombardment by a myriad sense impressions to which you are at every moment subjected. This withdrawal of attention from external objects affects all the senses. Bhramari Pranayama, Om sound and Yoni Mudra are useful for Pratyahara.
6. **Dharana (Concentration focussing of mind):** Fixing the mind on something is called Dharana. It may be outside or

inside. Concentration needs an inward turning of the mind. Awakening, serene mind, cheerfulness, regular practice of concentration, pranayama, celibacy, reduction of wants and activities, disciplined senses, Jap, control of anger, giving up reading novels, newspapers and watching T.V., are very helpful to develop the concentration capacity.

It calms the bubbling thoughts. Calm the surging emotions. Then alone you are able to concentrate. Concentrate on rising sun, moon, flower, picture of Lord Krishna, Rama, Buddha, Durga, Ista or picture of any saint. Practice twice a day atleast. Choose your concentration point according to your interest like—heart, eye brow centre, top of the head, nose, Muladhara etc.

7. **Dhyana (meditation):** Meditation is an unbroken flow of Dharana of the object is called Meditation. Meditation follows concentration, concentration merges in meditation. If you do meditation for half an hour daily, you can get mental peace and power, Divine energy, happiness, tension free mentality and doubtless mind.

Meditation kills all pains, sufferings and sorrows. It is the most powerful mental and nerve tonic. It provides spiritual strength. Meditation is the key to unlock many of the secrets of life. Meditation opens the door to intuitive knowledge and realms of eternal bliss. During practice of meditation you may feel as if a mysterious, inner voice is guiding you.

Mind wants a concrete object for meditation in the beginning. Meditate on Om, breath with the sound So-Ham After Sakshi dhyan meditate on Nirguna Brahama.

8. **Samadhi (Superconsciousness):** Samadhi is union with God. The state of Samadhi is beyond description. The state of Samadhi is all-bliss, joy and peace. In Samadhi the meditator

loses his individuality and becomes identical with the Supreme-Self. The meditator and the meditated object become one.

Faith, power of concentration of mind, memory for contemplation, celibacy and discernment (Pragya) are the means for the attainment of Samadhi. There are two types of Samadhi—Jad and Chaitanya Samadhi; Savikalpa and Nirvikalpa Samadhi or Asampragyata and Nirbeej Samadhi. You can get Kaivalya through Samadhi.

The first five limbs are external practices and last three (Sanyama) are internal practices of Raja Yoga. Eight Siddhies and Nav Niddhies are the results of Raja Yoga.

We will explain every part separately in details in the book.

• • •

6

Yama and Niyama

Yama

There are five 'Yamas'. Let us discuss here in brief.

1. Ahimsa

Ahimsa is not merely non-killing but a positive, cosmic love also. It is perfect harmless feeling and quality of the heart. It is Supreme love. Ahimsa is a weapon of the strong person. It can't be practised by weak persons. Ahimsa means to have 'no ill-will' what-so-ever, because oneself or Ataman dwells in all. All are manifestation of God.

There is no power greater than Ahimsa. It transmute man into Divinity. Ahimsa develops the soul-force or will-power and spiritual strength. Practice of Ahimsa should be done by mentally, verbally and in deed. Anger can be easily controlled by the practice of Ahimsa.

The mind must be freed from the thoughts of anger, jealousy, hatred, pride and egoism, one should entertain, thoughts of love, mercy, humility forgiveness, and forbearance in order to practise Ahimsa.

If you develop this one virtue, Ahimsa all other virtues will cling to you by themselves. If you have patience, forgiveness and self-control you can practise Ahimsa keeping away the insult, rebuke, censure and assault.

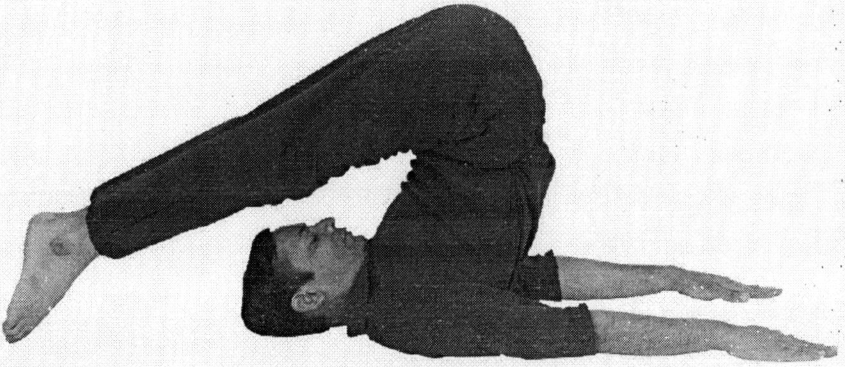

HALASANA

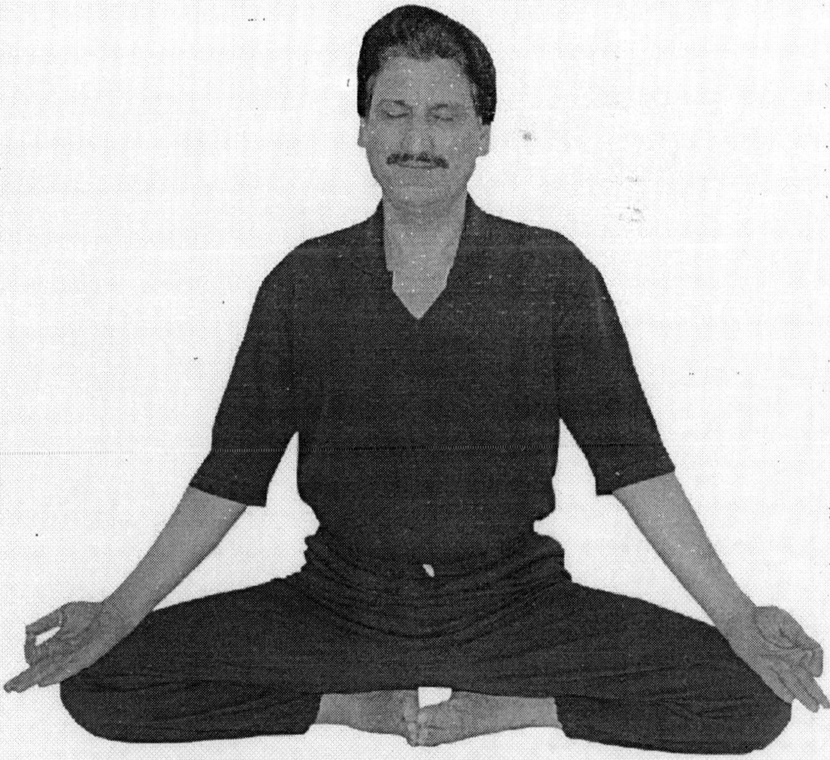

GORAKSHASANA

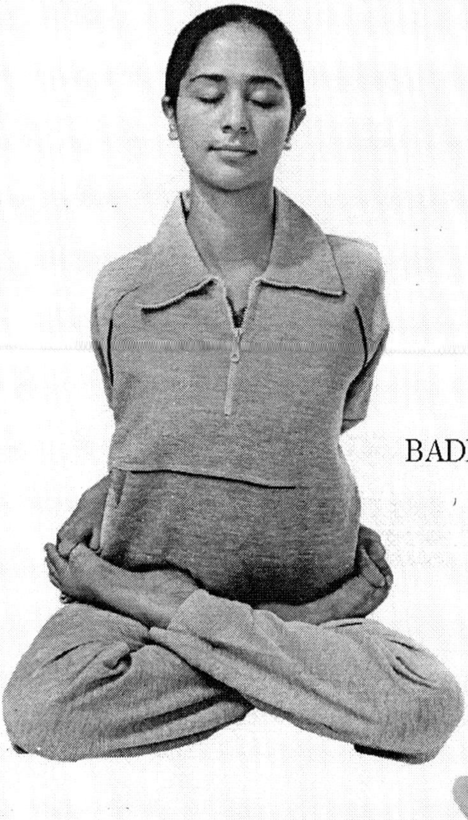

BADDHAPADMASANA

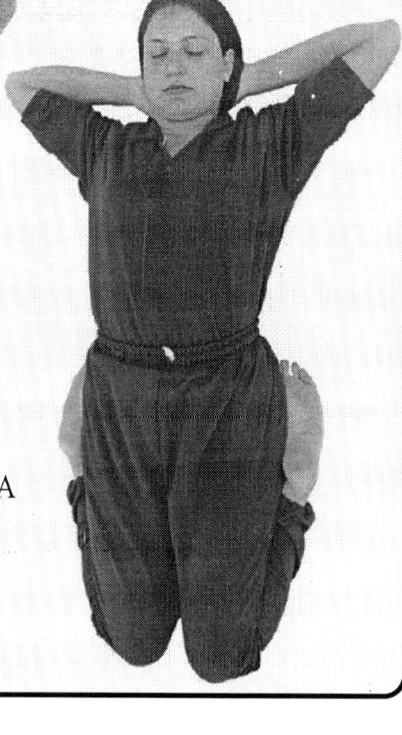

SUPTA VAJRASANA

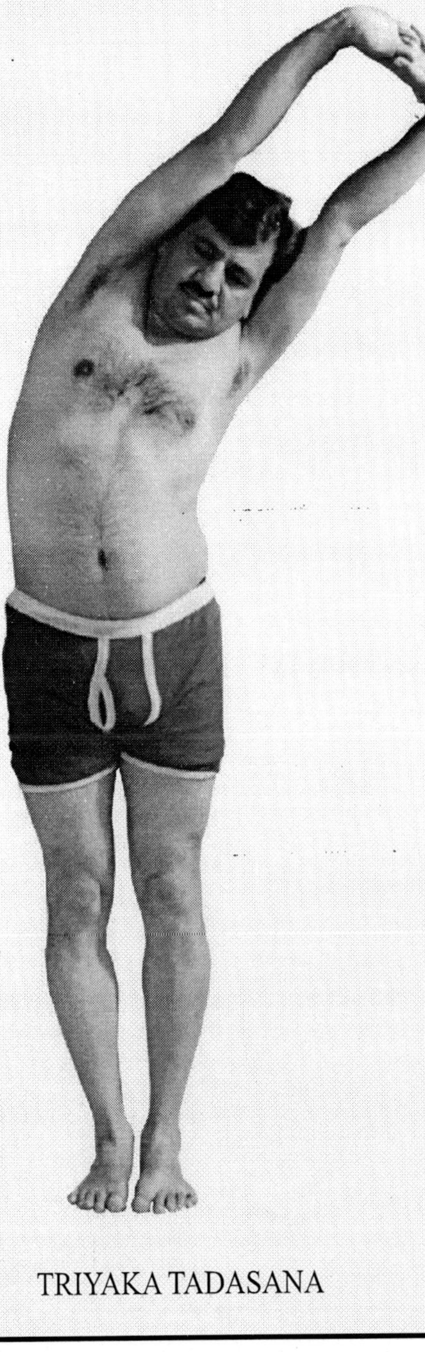

TRIYAKA TADASANA

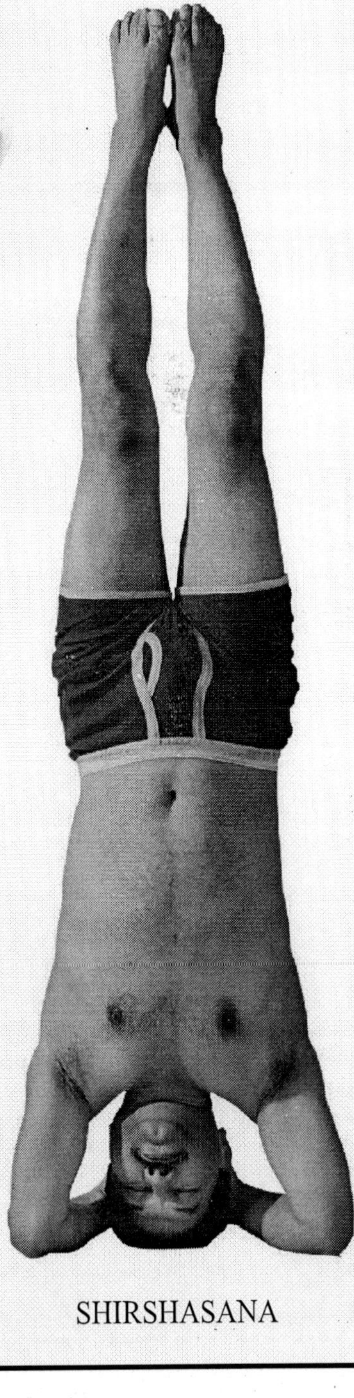

SHIRSHASANA

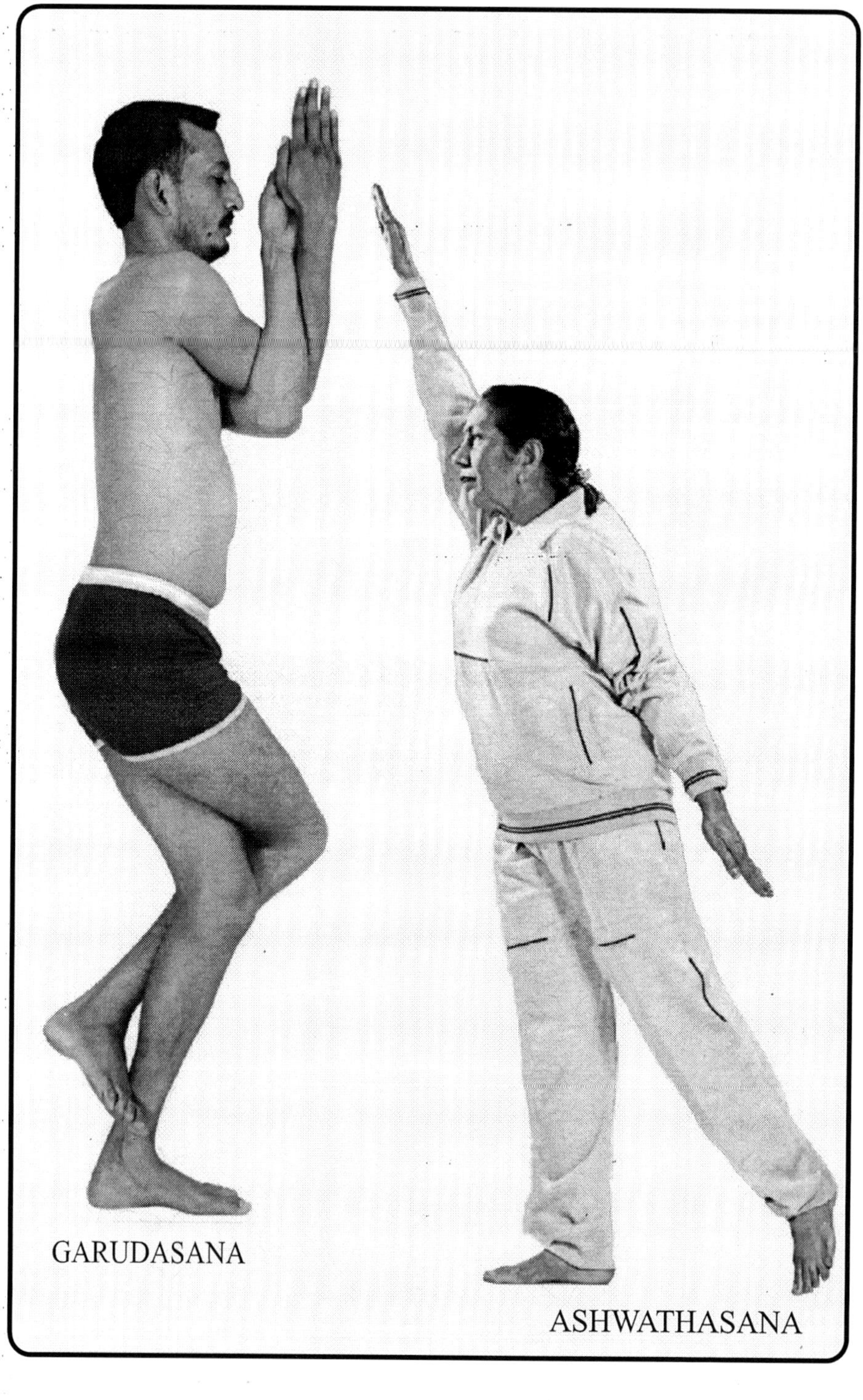

GARUDASANA

ASHWATHASANA

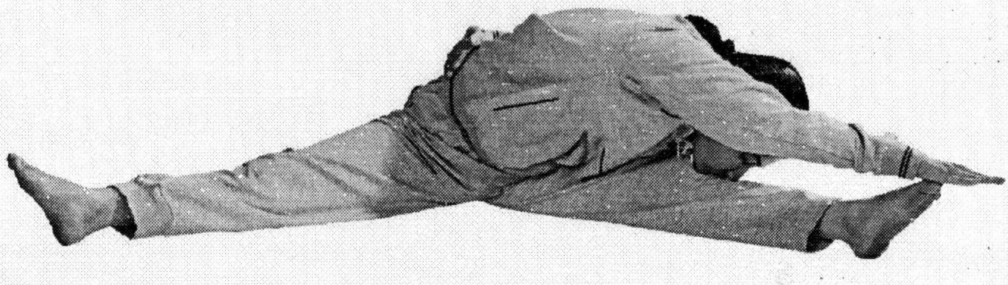

KAMAR CHAKRASANA

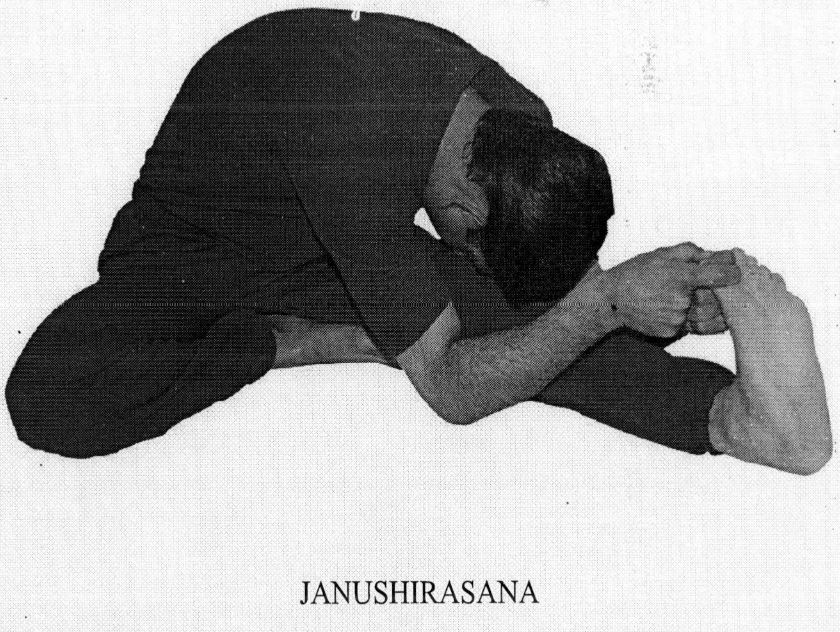

JANUSHIRASANA

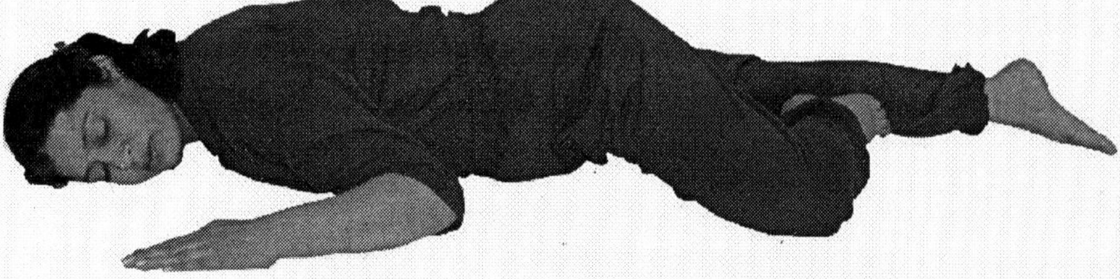

SHITHILASANA

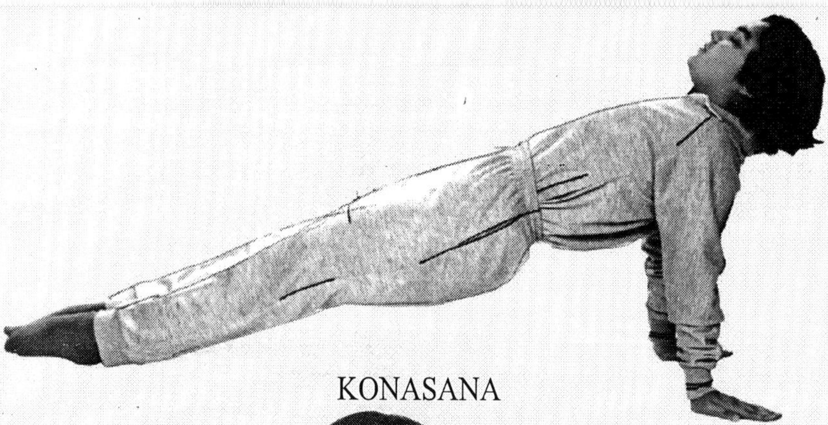

KONASANA

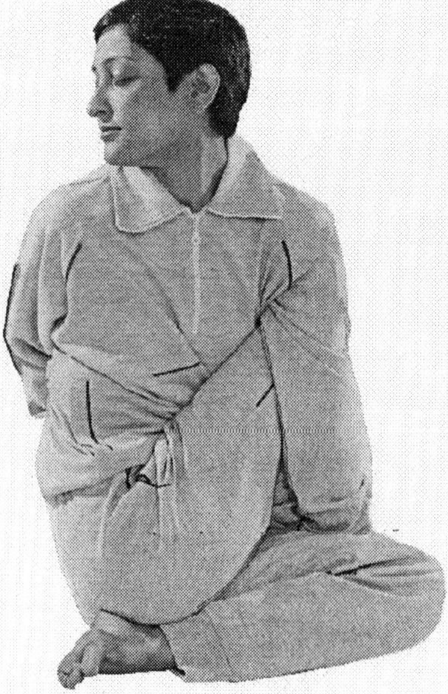

ARDHAMATSYENDRASANA

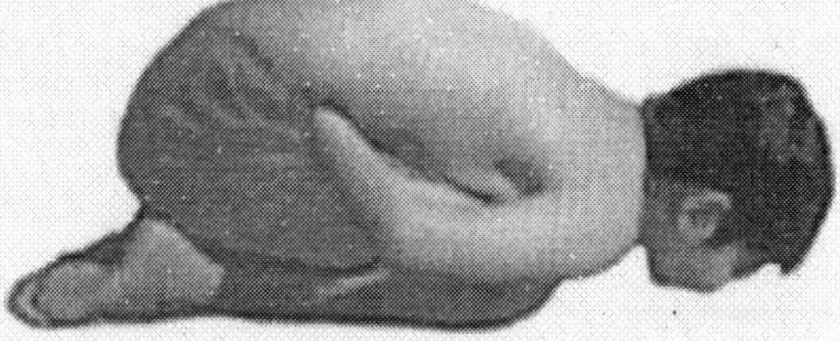

MANDUKASANA

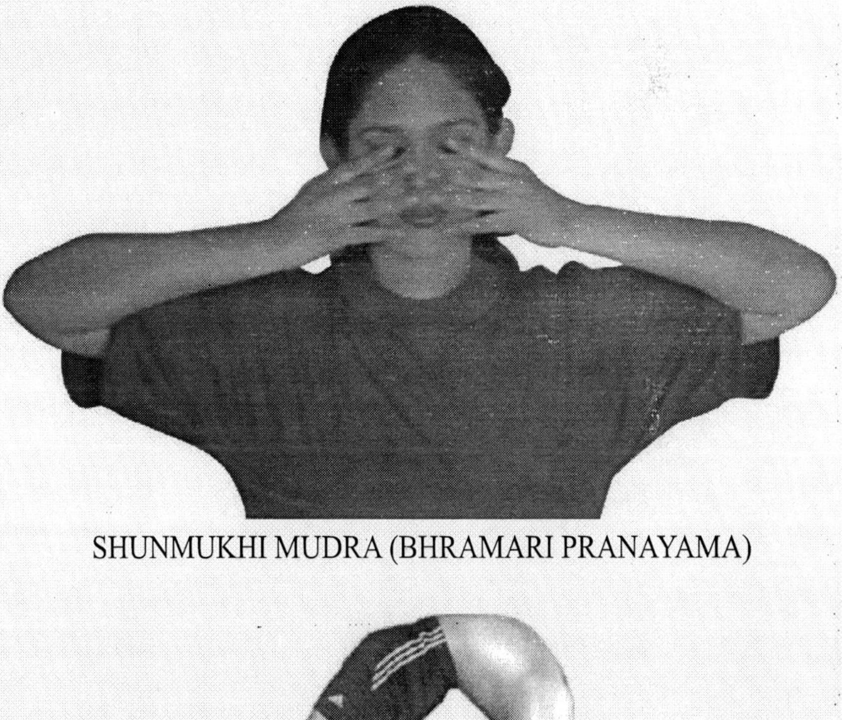

SHUNMUKHI MUDRA (BHRAMARI PRANAYAMA)

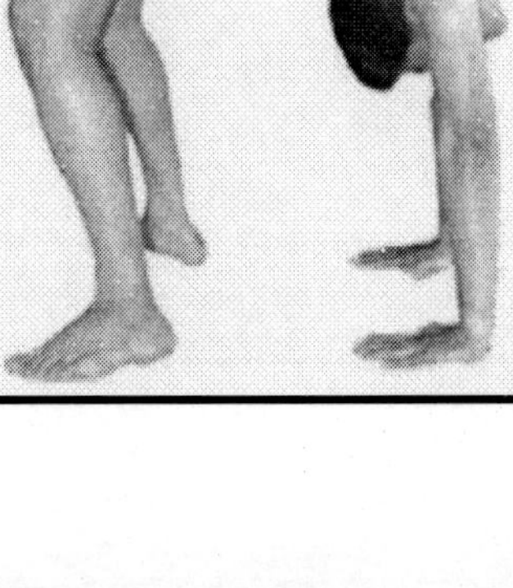

CHAKRASANA

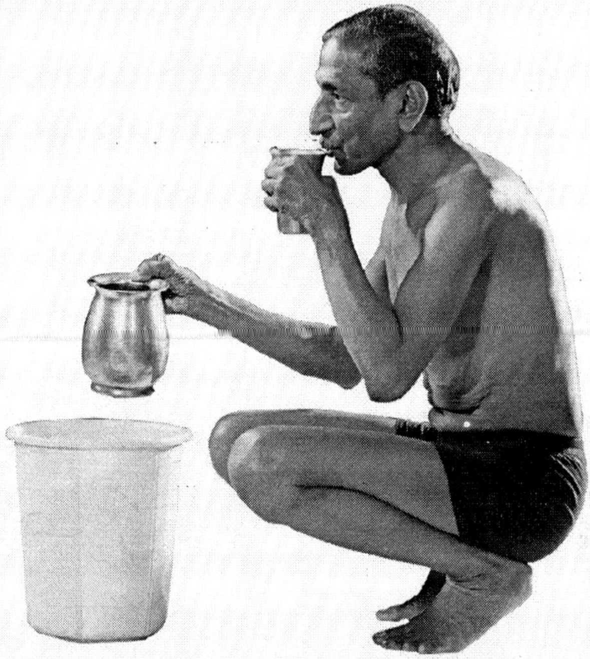

KUNJALA
I

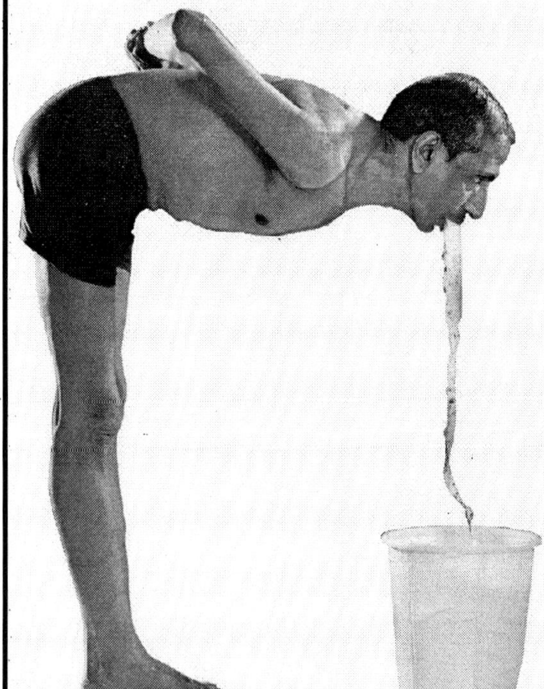

KUNJALA
II

2. Satya (Truthfulness)

Satya means being truthful in thought, speech and action. One should not exalt falsehood in thoughts words or action. Truth ultimately triumphs. Whatever you have seen or heard must he spoken of as it is. Don't twist or modify this, is Satya. To be true to one's own self is Satya. If you are established in truth, all other virtues will cling to you. By speaking truth the mind is purified, and the Divine light dawns. Ahimsa, Brahmcharya, purity, justice, harmony, forgiveness, peace, impartiality, self-control, modesty, endurance, goodness, renunciation, fortitude, compassion, are the forms of truth.

Mahatma Gandhi, King Harish Chandra and the great men-women are famous for their truthful attitude. Truthfulness is one of the three attributes of God, the other two being bliss and consciousness. Sadhaka of Truth gets respect from all.

Honesty and simplicity are two qualities that are a "must" for a yoga student and every individual in the society. Over come greed and ambition. Speak the truth lovingly, do not speak the truth which is harsh. Speaking the truth helps us to hear the voice of consciousness, augments confidence and self-reliance, removes complexes and bestows upon us the brilliant glow of truth in our faces.

3. Asteya (Non-stealing)

The meaning of Asteya is abstinence from stealing. It does not mean only taking away a thing that belongs to somebody else, wealth should be benefittingly used for public purpose. One should use money as a Divine gift. If we don't allow our surplus money to serve others in distress, it means we are stealing it from God. If we use wealth for social purpose, it becomes a '**meritorious activity**' and in the terminology of yoga, this meritorious behaviour is called Asteya.

Desire or want, greed, ambitions and the lack of discipline of the senses are the root cause of stealing.

Asteya is to be practised in thought, word and deed, one should acquire things by honest means and not by stealing, cheating or by resorting to dishonest and corrupt practices, otherwise peace of mind can never be acquired. Develop vairagya and love for all. Live simple life having least needs. If you are established in Asteya, all wealth will come to you. The habit of satisfaction can help in this matter.

4. Brahmcharya (Celibacy)

Brahmcharya is purity or freedom from lust in thought, word and deed. It is freedom from sexual thoughts, sexual urge and the attraction of sex. In other words controlling of senses and mind in word, deed and thought, is called Brahmcharya. Preserving of seminal energy and meditating on God constantly is real Brahmcharya.

Uncontrolled indulgence in sensual pleasures leads to many psychological disorders like mental deficiency, organic depression, fear complex, anxiety and irritation.

Brahmcharya elevates the mind and increases mental sharpness and alertness. By the conservation and sublimation of the sex-energy a yogi develops immense powers. Semen is the root cause of energy. Sadhana will make wonderful progress due to Brahmcharya.

Repression or suppression of sex-energy will not help in the practice of Brahmcharya. Think and feel that your wife and all other women are your mother or Blessed virgin Mary, mother of God.

Japa, Kirtan, Sattvic food, enquiry, yogasanas Padangusthasana utkatasana and siddhasana, pranayama (Nadishodhana) and meditation, will help you to get success in Brahmcharya. If you are established in Brahmcharya, you will have tremendous energy and gigantic will power.

Control your senses and mind. Don't discuss or think about love matter and about sex, a desire to be in the company of the other sex, are all forms of lust. Avoid the company of woman in solitude (akaant).

5. Aparigraha (Non-Avariciousness)

Aparigraha is freedom from greed or covetousness. Possession of wealth and property more than the basic need is called prigraha. It develops anxiety to preserve fear of loss, sorrow in loss, hatred, anger, untruthfulness, stealing, attachment, disappointment, agitation of mind, restlessness, cares and worries. Aprigraha removes all these and gives peace, contentment and satisfaction. It is an aid to the practice of Ahimsa, Satya and Asteya.

Aparigraha also specifically means non-receiving of gifts conducive of luxury. When a man does not receive present, his mind becomes pure. Live a simple life and save your time and energy for Sadhana. Non-greed is a very important spiritual quality. It is a great promoter of peace of mind. Aprigraha makes a person share the happy moments in the life even with strangers. We can learn the lesson from Nature. The sun, moon, air, river etc., don't hold or collect any thing. They go on giving and distributing. They are serving the world with selfless attitude, Vairagya, trustiship feelings, non-attachment and giving the extra wealth/money to needy in the society are very useful qualities in yoga life.

Niyama (Discipline, Observances)

There are five 'Niyamas' let us discuss here in brief.

1. Shouch (outer and inner cleanliness/purify)

This includes cleanliness of the body and the mind. A clean mind means a mind which is free of passions like greed, envy, jealousy, hatred, fear, egoism, attachment, tamas and rajas tendencies.

Yoga lays a clear cut emphasis on purity. It has laid down six process of eliminating impurities. It is known as ***Shatkarm***. These six processes are *Neti, Dhauti, Basti, Nauli, Trataka* and *Kapalbhati.* We will discuss these with curative aspect of this book.

The second variety of purity consists of keeping the whole mind free from six enemies. These are lust, anger, avarice, temptation, pride, vanity, false beliefs and ignorance. In a general sense, all the five yamas can be included under cleanliness of mind, because each one of them implies removal of some kind of impurity from the mind.

Selfless service, becoming positive thinker, loving all, doing good deeds, taking bath daily, weekly fasting, sattvic diet, control of food and sleep, control on senses and meditation are the means of purification. There is no achievement without purification of Chitta. So that it is very important Niyama.

2. Santosha (Contentment)

'*Santoshah Param Dhanam*' it is said in Hindu Shastras. We can reduce the desires due to Santosha. This satisfaction leads to power, happiness and peace. This is one of the striking qualities of a yogi who, in the absence of any idea of achievement or fulfilment of ambition, ever remains satisfied with whatever be confronts in life. So that we should satisfy from which we have gotten due to our purusartha (hard labout). We should minimise our needs and ambitions. When contentment comes, everything that belongs to this world becomes insignificant.

3. Tapas (Purificatory Action/austerity)

Tapas is purification of the mind, speach, senses and all actions that leads to the purification such as abstinence, fasting, duties, long Sadhana etc., are all under Tapas. The control of sense-organs, body and mind is austerity. Due to Tapas our great saints have got highest attainments. Tapas means a regular and long practice. We develop our capacity, tolerance power, will power, confidence Sidhies and equanimity of the mind.....

4. Swadhyaya (Self-study and study of scriptures)

Swadhyaya is the study of self-study of holi books and repetition of the Lord's name. To know one's own self is self-study. This process starts with self-introspection, with the study of scriptures and listening to the sermons of the saints, rishis and realised souls. It ensures both progress and pleasure. Study of the auto-biography is also helpful in Swadhyaya to get inspiration and awareness. Many problems related to Sadhana can be removed by Swadhyaya. It fills the mind with good and pious thoughts, and makes it peaceful....

5. Ishwara Pranidhana (Surrender to God)

This means relying on the Divine will, accepting every thing as the will of God. Through self-surrender comes Samadhi or superconsciousness state. It is a unique state of the mind. It is completely free from ego and pride. Sadhak dedicates every thing movable and immovable, thoughts, feelings and deeds to God. His mind becomes totally free from worldliness. He gets *Sahaja Awastha* of mind.

The Yamas and Niyamas are the basic steps of eight-fold ladder of Astanga yoga. Without the practice of Yamas and Niyamas one can't be succeed in Sadhana......

• • •

7

Yogasana

What is Yogasana?

'Asana' in Sanskrit means 'Posture of body' and 'yoga' means 'the Science of deep and subtle phenomenon of human awareness and organic functions. So, yogasana—different bodily postures, by which we can control, conduct, regularise and stimulate different organic and glandular functions of human body and its magnetic and cosmic force.

Importance of Yogasanas

- Yogasanas are far superior to the physical exercise because they are based on the detailed and all round study of human body as well as human awareness.
- They effect the glandular and pranic functions of the body, and thus resulting in the inner transformations of human personality.
- They develop physical, mental and spiritual efficiency.
- Awakening of pranic forces in the body intensifies the awareness, and thus, the higher unexplored centres of brain are harnessed. So, yogasanas, if done properly with full precautions and scientifically give astonishing results.
- Body becomes flexible, supple and elastic.

- Yogasanas do **'oiling'** in the various parts of the body and mind, ensures a smooth running and efficient working of the psychosomatic machine.
- Yogasanas are not just simple exercises but sustained, scientific, patterns of posture.
- In yogasanas the movement of the limbs has to be of a slow, spontaneous, uniformed nature, with no jerks at all.
- The neuro-muscular system is so composed that for every group of muscles that go into contraction, another group undergoes relaxation.
- Yogasanas, by their very nature recognise and recondition, the system, to bring about physiological harmony between the two.
- According to the classics, the object of the yogasanas is to provide stability and well-being ('Sthira Sukham Asanam')
- Yogasanas are the physical techniques, they make the body and its organs strong. They build not only muscles and bones but they make all the systems strong enough to keep themselves to perfect health.
- They check the high rate and speed of decay of the body tissues. Energy is generated. The loss incurred due to exertion and worry of the world, is made by the practice of yogasanas.
- Yogasanas provide freshness, adaptability, agility etc.
- Yogasanas make the mind strong and cultivate will power, develop strong determination, perseverance and equilibrium.
- Sadhaka does not become upset by trifling disturbances that come in course of daily life.
- Life becomes easy, natural, growing and flowing. Difficulties do not seem to be difficulties at all.

- Yogasanas are not to be taken as physical activities alone but they are Yogic Kriyas as well, deviced to develop the latent powers of man.
- Yogasanas help to make the latent glands active, the man becomes powerful in speech, behaviour and action like Sri Aurobindo, Vivekananda, Dayananda, Maharshi Raman, Swami Shivananda, Tulsidas, Sooardas etc.
- Kundalani yogins, Hatha yogins, Tantra yogins and modern theological sects of today have accepted the value of yogasanas.
- Yogasanas have become very popular in the present age in Bharat and in western countries both for their psycho physiological advantages.
- Their reputation for therapeutic values have now been highly acclaimed in the field of medicine and therapy. There are yoga departments in big hospitals. Every body must practise yogasanas daily.
- Yogasanas are published in magazines and news paper. T.V. channels are showing regular programmes about yogasanas.
- In other systems of physical exercise, the internal organs of the body don't get proper exercise while yogasanas give sufficient massage to the inner parts.
- There is no expenditure in doing yogasanas. They have no need of additional foods for practising.
- Yogasanas are helpful to purify the body and mind.
- Yogasanas increase the life span.
- Yogasanas are called "**non-violent activity**'. Yogasanas require the least possible energy.

Difference between yogasanas and Exercises

Body Exercise	Yogasanas
1. The body becomes stiff due to unnatural pressure.	1. The body becomes elastic
2. Glands are not evenly influenced.	2. The glands secrete their juices in regulated manner.
3. The waste matter is not dispelled.	3. The entire waste matter is excreted by the arteries.
4. Breathing activity becomes erratic.	4. Owing to the control over the breathing activity, we reap many benefits of inhalation and exhalation at the physical and mental level. Moreover our lungs become strong.
5. Outward muscles are exercised.	5. Internal organs are as much influenced as the external.
6. Very often; our digestive system becomes weak because the supply of blood does not reach those parts of the body due to the brisk activity in other parts.	6. The regular blood circulation in our entire body systematises the digestive matizes the digestive system in toto.
7. It is only the physical body that is influenced.	7. The astral body is influenced along with the physical. More importantly one gains control over the mind.
8. One does not develop any kind of seminal control.	8. The practice of yogasanas results in the preservation of semen and its upward movement.

9. There is a possibility of an awkward development of the body.	9. The all round body development in a regulated manner enhances our beauty and health. The body becomes sound, calm and the face lustrous.
10. The physical exercise can never ensure a complete cure of diseases.	10. Ailments do not come near and longevity is natural consequence.
11. Intellectual development that sublimates human life can never be possible.	11. Yogasanas are instrumental in the development of such invaluable virtues as tolerance, steadfastness, self-restraint and self-confidence.
12. Lack of concentration and proper judgement in practical life.	12. Concentration and introversion reform practical life. Positive thoughts replace the negative ones.
13. Physical exercise causes fatigue.	13. Yogasanas relieve the fatigue and make the body light and active.
14. Both time and our vital energy are wasted away.	14. Lesser energy is spent in lesser time. As a result not only more benefits are reaped but vital energy is also well preserved.
15. Old and weak people are incapable of doing every kind of exercise.	15. Every person a child of eight or an old man can do yogasanas. Weak person can do with the permission of yoga expert.

16. Open space and many things and gadgets are needed.	16. There is no need of any aids, only a little space is enough.
17. Sports and exercises cannot be possible during journey.	17. Yogasanas can be performed even while undertaking journey.
18. It is an individual benefit phenomenon.	18. Yogasanas have their social-impacts.

Important Directions about Yogasanas

To take the full advantage of yogasanas, it is advisable to follow the following directions and principles.

1. The first principle of yogic postures is that they should be practised in a slow and steady manner, and all kinds of jerks should be carefully avoided.
2. The second principle is that having attained a final position in a particular posture, one should maintain the posture in a comfortable and relaxed manner.
3. While maintaining the posture one should concentrate on the relaxed muscles and try to relax them further, mind should not be allowed to wander.
4. The fourth principle is that in attaining or maintaining the final position in any of the postures, due regard should be given to limitations set by one's age, sex and bodily condition.
5. The fifth principle is to reap the maximum benefit from the yogasanas, the practice should be regular, uninterrupted, and performed with full conviction.
6. Asanas should be selected according to the individual state of health, abnormality and capacity.
7. For the prescription of Asanas for oneself, a yoga teacher should be consulted, who has a perfect knowledge of physiology, anatomy, flow of prana, and also psychology.

8. Number and duration of yogasanas should be gradually increased.
9. Yogasanas should be prac tised in the morning before taking breakfast and afte : clearing the bowels.
10. Diet, sleep and rest should be adjusted so as to avoid constipation, for subtle benefits.
11. Yogasanas should be practised in open park, lawn. If you do in a room, that should be clean, ventilated (but without heavy air flow). To avoid accidents keep away the fire, instruments, machines, fan, chair, etc., near you.
12. The carpet for yogasanas should not be much soft to avoid slips. There should be no bare floor ground to practise the yogasanas. A thick blanket must be used.
13. Take sufficient rest after every yogasana. Lie down in shavasna; even between doing yogasanas whenever one feels tired.
14. Don't take bath immediately after yogasanas. Bath should be taken at least 15 minutes before yogasanas, or half an hour thereafter.
15. After half an hour of yogasanas, one may take milk, fruit, dalia, sprouted cereal or some light and natural breakfast.
16. For spiritual benefits, each posture should be done very slowly and for a longer time.
17. Inverted postures like sarvangasana or sheershasana must be performed in the end, to avoid harms and to get better results and toning of the brain.
18. Clothing, should be in accordance with the season, and loose clothes are preferred. Save yourself from cold in winter.
19. One should remain silent while practising yogasanas. Keep the eyes closed throughout the practice.

20. Concentrate on breath, chakra and on the limbs which have a stress. Concentration in the practice of yogasanas is necessary for the all round progress of the body and the mind.
21. There should be a gradual increase in the time duration in the practice of yogasanas. Body becomes flexible in a short time. It will easily accomplish a perfect state in each yogasana.
22. Before going to the final state the basic steps should be properly practised.
23. Remember slow and rhythmic breathing is the key to concentration and relaxation.
24. There should be 3 hours gap between meal and practice of yogasanas.
25. Never practise to the stage of exhaustion. Remember pain is a signal to stop.
26. While performing asanas, the breathing should be smooth and normal and always through the nose. When you bend forward in any yogasana, you exhale. When your body stretches backward or straightens out, you inhale. It is a bellows. When you want to go on bending further, take small breaths. When you apply force in bending or balancing the body, the breath should be held for a few seconds.
27. When you do a yogasana with one leg/arm, do it with the other too.
28. Relax the body and have normal breathing after each yogasana.
29. Don't attempt Shirshasana (Head stand pose) without proper guidance from a yoga teacher.

30. In standing postures, always keep your eyes open.
31. If you are practising a yogasana to relieve a specific disease or weakness, hold it for longer than usual, and practise it more often.
32. When the asana becomes perfect, don't repeat it, just increase the time it is held initially, however, do each asana two or three times.
33. No undue strain should be felt in the facial muscles, ears, eyes or in breathing during the practice of yogasanas.
34. If you are suffering from complicated diseases or severe fever, don't practise asanas.
35. Women should not practice asanas four months after conception and for three months after delivery and during menstruation.
36. Begin your yogasanas by reciting or chanting Ganesh/Saraswati/Gayatri/Om three times, thus you have prepared your body and mind for an ideal practice of yoga.
37. If you have a fractured bone, you should not practice difficult yogasanas, otherwise the bone may break again at the same place.
38. Conclude your yogasanas with prayer for peace and harmony in the world. Fill your mind with positive and elevated thoughts for yourself and for humanity. You may conclude your 'abhyasa' with the long chants of Om.

Special Hints

1. Yogasanas are not only scientific exercises but also have the tremendous results. Yogasanas should be done either in empty stomach or only after three hours of taking food. Morning time is the best time.

2. Ladies are not advised to do yogasanas during menstrual period and difficult yogasanas in case of pregnancy after three months.
3. Blood pressure patient and heart patient should do yogasanas only with yogacharya's advice.
4. Don't do yogasanas when you feel tired, weak and when you didn't have proper sleep the previous night.
5. Take rest after every yogasana, normalise your breathing.
6. Do yogasanas in open air, at silent and clean place according to your capacity. Use carpet/gadda to do asanas.
7. The yogasanas are for health making, preventive, and curative, they increase resistance, endurance and will power. There are five types of yogasanas as—meditative poses, standing, sitting, poses, on belly poses and on spineposes.

Names of the Asanas in Sanskrit and English

Original Name	English Name
1. Shirshashana	Topsy-Turvy pose Head Stand
2. Bhujangasana	Cobra Pose
3. Shalbhasana	Lucust Pose
4. Dhanurasana	Bowpose
5. Halasana	Plow Pose
6. Sarvangasana	Shoulder Stand Pose
7. Matsyasana	Fish Pose
8. Vipareet Karani	Pelvic Pose
9. Paschi-mottanasana	Back Stretching Pose
10. Ardha-Matsyendrasana	Spine-Twisting Pose
11. Yoga Mudra	Psychic Union Pose Colon-Toning Pose, Symbol of Yoga

12. Shavasana	Corpse Pose
13. Padmasana	Lotus Pose
14. Siddhasana	Accomplished Pose
15. Padhastasana	Standing Posterior Stretch
16. Mayurasana	Peacock Pose
17. Vajrasana	Thuderbolt Pose Adamant Pose
18. Baddha Padmasana	Adept Posture Locked Lotus Pose
19. Kukkutasana	Cock Posture
20. Uttankurmasana	Tortoise Posture
21. Parbatasana	Mountain Posture
22. Chakrasana	Wheel Posture
23. Trikonasana	Triangle Posture
24. Janusirasana	Knee head Posture
25. VrischiKasana	Scorpion Pose
26. Padottanasana	Raised legs Pose
27. Pawan Muktasana	Leg lock Pose
28. Naukasana	Boat Pose
29. Udrakarshasana	Abdomial Stretch Pose
30. Makarasana	Crocodile Pose
31. Sukhasana	Easy Pose
32. Swastikasana	Auspicious Pose
33. Simhasana	Lion Pose
34. Veerasana	Hero's Pose
35. Marjari	Cat Pose
36. Shashankasana	Hare/Moon Pose
37. Ustrasana	Camel Pose
38. Suptvajrasana	Sleeping Thunder bolt pose
39. Tadasana	Palm Tree Pose
40. Surya Namaskara	Salutations to the Sun
41. Garbhasana	Womb Pose

42.	Kandhasana	Shoulder Pose
43.	Konasana (Setu)	Bridge Pose
44.	Gomukhasana	Cow's Face Pose
45.	EK Pad Pranamasana	One legged Prayer Pose
46.	Natrajanasana	Lord Shiva's Pose
47.	Pad angusthanasana	Tiptop Pose
48.	Akaran Dhanurasana	Archer's Pose
49.	Gorakshasana	Yogi Gorakhnath's Pose
50.	Balasana	Pose of the child

Classification of Yogasanas

The classification of Yogasanas can be done in many ways. Here they have been divided in four groups:

1. Static and Dynamic Poses.
2. Meditative and Curative (cultural) Poses.
3. Sitting, Standing, Abdominal, Spinal, Hand and Head Poses.
4. Groupwise.

Swami Satyanand Saraswati classified them in three groups:

A. **The Beginners Group:**
   - Pawan Muktasana Series 1, 2, 3
   - Meditative Asanas
   - Vajrasana Group of Asanas
   - Standing Asanas

B. **The Intermediate Group:**
   - Padmasana Group Asanas
   - Backward Bending Asanas
   - Forward Bending Asanas
   - Side Twisting Asanas
   - Inverted Asanas
   - Balancing Asanas

C. **Advance Group:**
   - Difficult Asanas.

Methods and Benefits of Yogasanas

There are about 84 yogasanas, which are very useful and effective, the main yogasanas are given below:

1. Suryanamaskara

Suryanamaskara is accompanied by regulation and has 12 steps.

Method: Stand erect with the legs and palms together.

1. Take the hands together at chest height. Breathe normally.
2. Raise your arms slowly above the head; move them backward, and your head too (ears should be within your stretched arms); Breathe in deeply.
3. Bend your body forward very slowly. Your palms should touch the ground either side of your feet. Your legs must remain straight. Exhale fully.

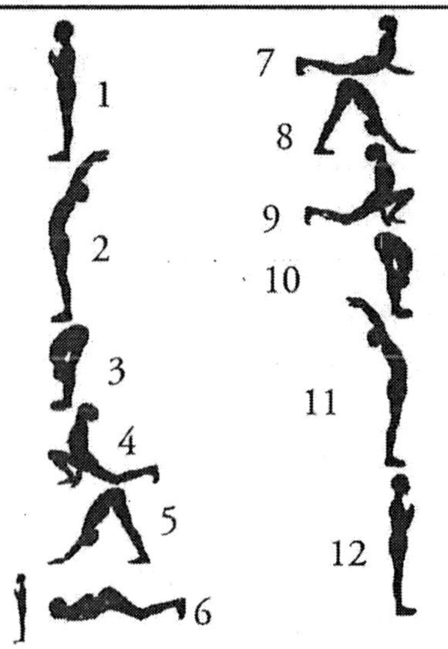

Surya Namaskar

Fig. 1

4. Slowly stretch your right leg backward still the knee touches the ground look up and inhale. Touch the thigh with the heel.

5. Stretch the left leg gently backward; support yourself your stretched arms and toes at 30° Exhale fully.
6. Bend at the knee and rest the knees on the floor without altering the positions of the palms and toes. Rest the forehead on the ground. Breathe normally. The buttocks will be raised up.

   Fore head, palms, knees and toes, all the eight organs will be touching the ground.
7. Inhale, raise the head and trunk making the spine concave upward without changing the position, the legs and pelvis remain on the ground.
8. Exhale, raise the buttocks up. Keep the head inward, have a complete arch, with the heels and palms touching the ground.
9. Inhale, bring the right leg forward between the palms and in line with them. Arch the back concave as in step 4.
10. 10, 11 &12 the last three positions are the same as positions 3, 2 & 1.

Benefits:

- It contributes to muscular strength, feeling of endurance as well as exhilaration.
- It makes spine and limbs flexible.
- It develops the breathing capacity. It reduces the abdominal fat etc.

2. Padmasana

Method: Padmasanas represent Lotus. Sit on the ground spreading the legs forward. Then place the right foot on the left thigh and the left foot on the right thigh. Place the hands on the knee-joints in Gyanmudra or Brahmanjali.

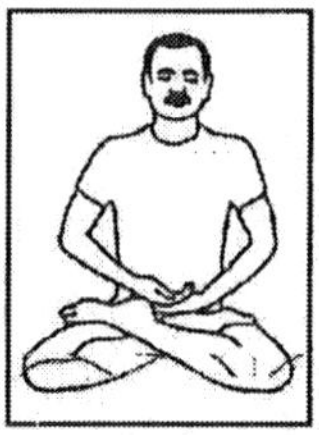

Fig. 2

Benefits:

- It gives relaxation, purity, sublimity of the mind.
- It improves memory and concentration.
- It makes the spinal column flexible.
- It improves digestion, expands chest, corrects ailments of heart and mind, corrects the arthritis.
- It helps in celibacy.
- It strengthens the lungs.

3. Vajrasana

Method: Sit with legs extended and together, bending the knees one by one and put the legs under the buttocks with toes pointing inward. Put the palms on the knees and the knees close together, sit comfortably. Keep the spine erect, eyes closed, the body relaxed concentrate on your breathing.

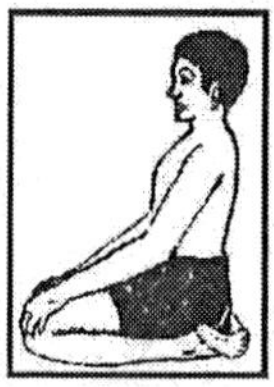

Fig. 3

Benefits:

- It is only asana which can be performed with a full belly.
- It improves digestion.
- It helps in dyspepsia, constipation, colitis, seminal weakness and in easing the stiffness of the legs.
- It corrects ailments of thigh, abdomen, caves, spinal column and lumber region.

4. Supt Vajrasana

Method: Sit in Vajrasana. Keeping the legs a bit apart put your buttock on the ground. Supporting the elbow lie down on the ground backward. Keep your folded arms under your head. Take rest, come back on Vajrasana with the help of your elbows and holding the ankles.

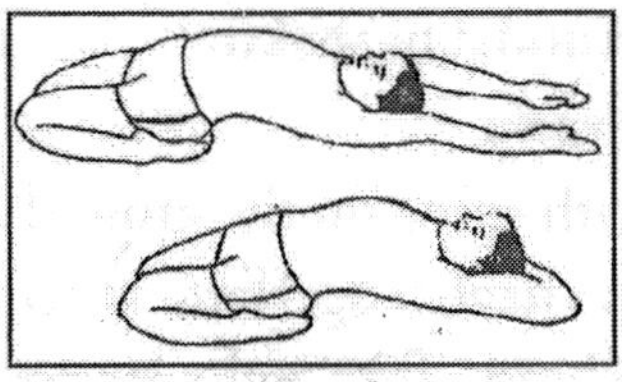

Fig. 4

Benefits:

- It corrects the disorders of the stomach, intestine, liver, kidneys, spleen and all the organs of the abdominal area.
- The ailments of spine and joints are effectively corrected by this asana.
- It enhances sexual potentiality.
- It removes indigestion, wind trouble, constipation and piles also.

5. Yogamudra

Method: Sit in Padmasana or Vajrasana. Place the fists backward near the catch the lumber region left fist from right hand. Inhale, bend slowly down breathing out from lumber region. Your forehead and nose touch the ground.

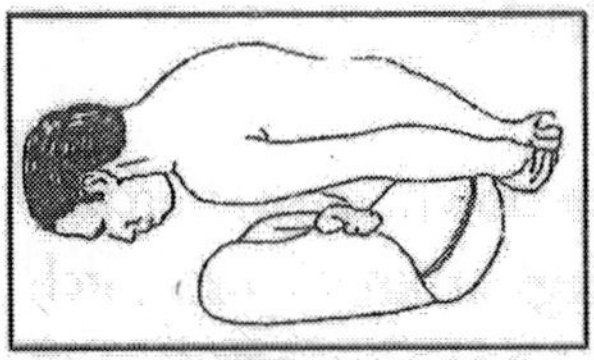

Fig. 5

Exhale the breath and stay as long as you can. Come up slowly and breathe in

Benefits:

- Corrects ailments of hands, legs, lumber and back.
- Helps in proper development of these parts.

- Strengthens chest and lungs.
- Helps in correcting tonsilitis and asthma.
- Purifies mind, improves concentration and intellect.
- It activates Kundalini shakti.

6. Pawana Muktasana

Method: Lie with spine on the ground over a blanket/dari, heels together, arms stretched above the head. Take right leg to 45° position. Keep the knee straight. Inhale, bend the knee. Press it on the chest by the interlocked fingers. Exhale, touch your nose to the knee. Come in normal position and inhale. Repeat this by the left leg and with the both legs. Roll right and left five times.

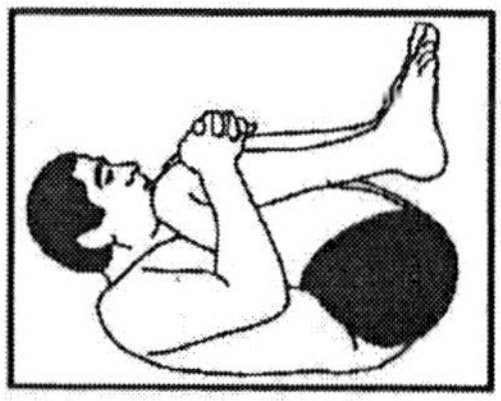

Fig. 6

Benefits:

- Helps to remove gaseous accumulations in the stomach and constipation.
- Improves the spread of back and shoulders.
- Straightens the spinal column removing the displacements, defects, if any.
- Corrects ailments of lumber region, legs, hands, head and ribs.
- Relieves backache.

7. Dhanurasana

Method: Lie face down, arms stretched in front. Bend the legs at knees and catch the ankles with corresponding hands. Lift the knees and thighs off the ground. Simultaneously, inhale and raise the head and chest until you are poised on abdomen, slowly come back, put legs and chest on the ground, take rest and relax the body.

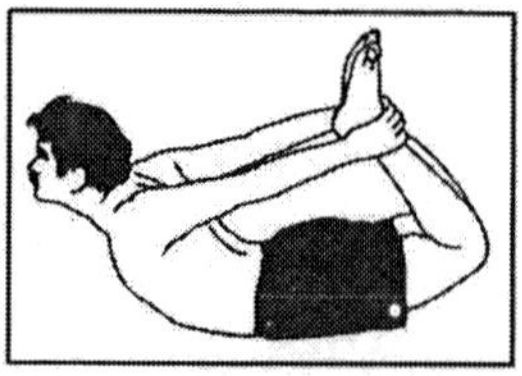

Fig. 7

Benefits:

- It corrects ailments of spinal column, neck, lumber, hands, legs, abdomen and chest.
- It cures gastro intestinal ailments, dysentery.
- It improves digestion system.
- It removes obesity and diabetes.
- Dharan sets in its original position.

8. Paschimottanasana

Method: Sit down with stretched legs. Raise the hands over the head. Bend forward slowly till the head is on the knees and catch hold of the toes with respective hands. Remain in that position for some time. Breathe normally. Come back inhaling and stretching the arms.

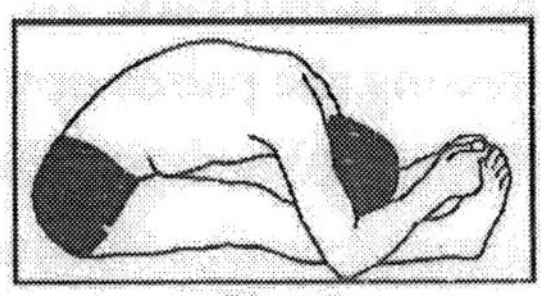

Fig. 8

Benefits:

- Corrects piles and diabetes.
- It improves the spinal column, legs, muscles and stomach tone.
- It cures gastro intestinal ailments, dysentery.
- Height is gained, waist line is trimmed.
- Constipation is removed.

9. Konasana

Method: Sit down with stretched legs together. Put the soles of the feet on the ground. The palms of the hands may be put behind yourself on the ground in such a manner that the fingers are pointed outward. Balance the body on the palms

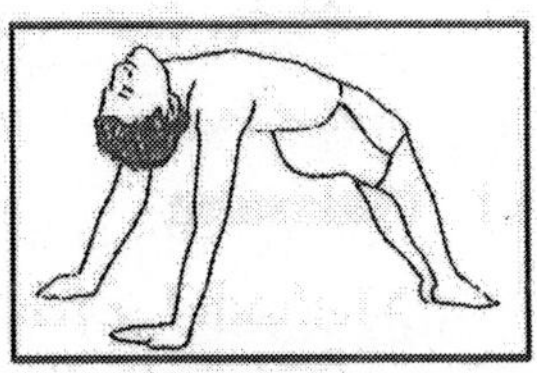

Fig. 9

and feet. Inhale and raise the navel and body upward. Normalise the breath. Exhaling and touching the chin to the chest, return slowly to the original position and rest.

Benefits:

- It is the counter pose of paschimottanasana.
- The digestive systems, excretory system and nervous system become healthy.
- It strengthens shoulders and wrists.
- It removes the diseases of spinal cord.

10. Sarvangasana

Method: Lie flat on the back, stretching both hands, the palms should be downward. Keep the legs together. Lift the legs pressing the palms upto 45°. Stay steady for a while and then raise the legs to a 60° angle, and proceed further till the legs reach a 90° angle, finally raise the trunk and legs till your body becomes vertical. Now keep your body steady for a few seconds or minutes. Come back slowly.

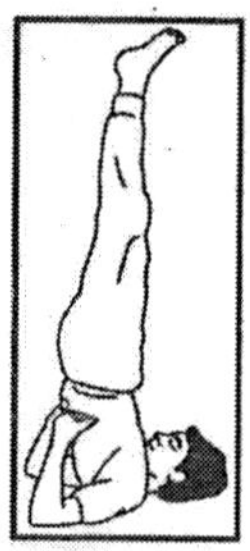

Fig. 10

Benefits:

- It keeps the thyroid healthy.
- Beneficially influences the pelvic organs, both in males and females.
- It is useful in curing varicose veins, piles, menstrual disorders.
  Note: Persons with cervical spondylitis should not do this asana.

11. Halasana

Method: Lie flat on the back, stretch the arms beside the body, palms turned downward. Keep the legs stiff and raise them up bringing them beyond the head gradually; bend the back well and try to touch the ground with the toes. Avoid bending the knees. Let the chin be well-pressed against the chest. Remain in this position for a while and then return slowly in the original position without raising the head.

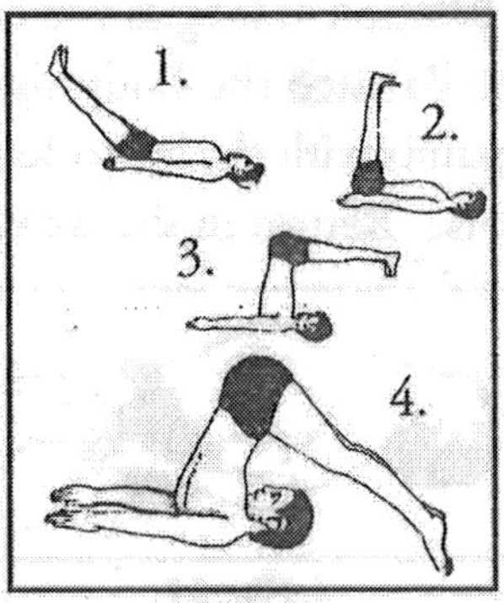

Fig. 11

Breathe-in while raising the legs. Breath-out while the legs are lowered to rest on the ground.

Benefits:

- It cures paralysis, rheumatism, sprain, spine ailments.
- Improves and functioning of the liver and endocrine glands.
- Corrects acidity, diabetes, flatulence, hydrocele and hernia.
- Maintains youthfulness and thyroid problems removes.

12. Tolungulasana

Method: Sit in Padmasana. Then lie on the back with padmasana intact. Put fists of both hands below the buttocks in the central position. Lift the head and knees to straight line. Duration three minutes.

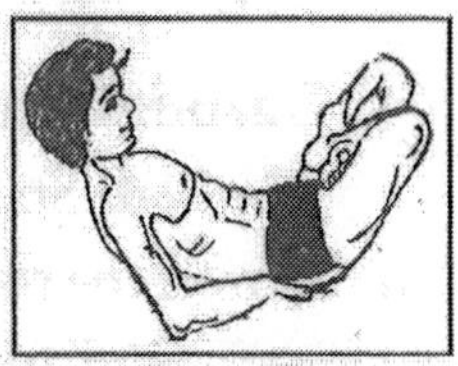

Fig. 12

Benefits:

- It Removes constipation and intestinal gases.
- Corrects obesity, kidney ailments and expands chest.
- Hand and Leg muscles become strong and supple.

13. Matsyasana

Method: Sit in Padmasana. Bend backwards until the back of your head touches the ground. Hold your big toes in your hands and supporting yourself on your head and the knees. Raise your back up. Stay in this position as long as you can. Then slowly regain the former position. Balance the body opon the buttocks, and elbows, and put the palms with the buttocks. Rotate the neck clock wise and anty clockwise. Return in shavasana.

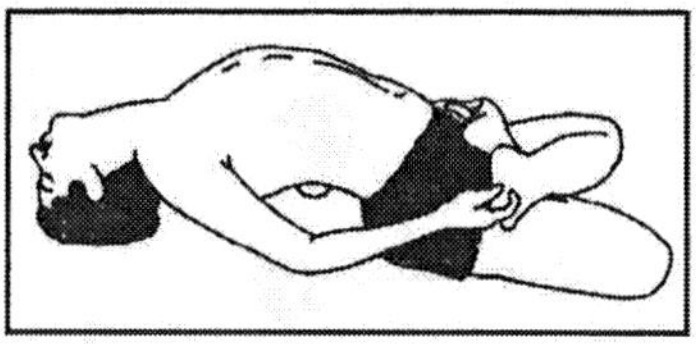

Fig. 13

Benefits:

- Corrects asthma, bronchitis and other lungs disorders.
- Expands chest.
- Improves digestion.
- Removes acidity, constipation, diabetes, eye diseases, tonsils, and other throat ailments.
- It prevents hair decay.
- It can bring the displaced navel back to its proper position.
- It regulates the menstrual cycle.

14. Garudasana

Method: Stand bending a little in knees. Cross one leg over the thigh of the other leg, twining the legs as shown. Similarly entwine the hands. Repeat it with other side.

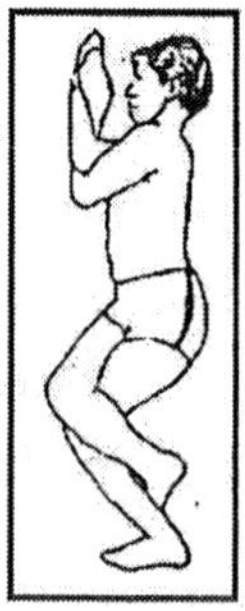

Fig. 14

Benefits:

- Correct inguinal, scrotal, uterine and vaginal hernia.
- It corrects hydrocele.

- It strengthens leg muscles. It is beneficial for those who work in standing pose/or walk much.

15. Ardha-Matsyendrasana

Method: Sit and stretch the legs. Bend the left knee and fix the heel at the perineum. Bend the right leg keeping the knee up and putting the sole on the outside of the left thigh. Twist the trunk as shown in the diagram to the right and press left hand around the right knee catching in line with the shoulder. Take the left hand from behind the back and place the right palm on left thigh. Maintain this posture and relax. Unfold slowly and come to the original position. Again start with right leg the whole process.

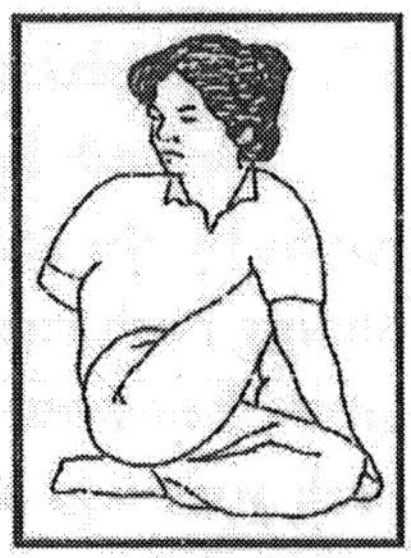

Fig. 15

Benefits:

- Build a healthy and elastic spinal column.
- It removes abdominal congestion Dyspepsia constipation, enlarged and congested liver and spleen, sluggish liver and inactive kidneys are put in a better condition.
- It is the best asana for diabetes.

16. Bhujangasana

Method: Lie down prone with legs stretched. Place the palms close to the chest parallel to the body. Raise the head, neck and the chest gradually together. Let the navel be touching the ground. Remain for a few seconds in this posture with inhaling. Come back with exhaling. Take rest and repeat again.

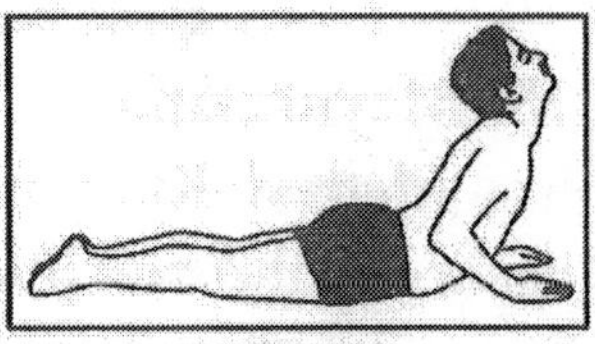

Fig. 16

Benefits:

- It is useful in cervical spondylitis, kyphosis, asthma, bronchitis and backaches.

- It corrects ailments of hands, semen, spinal column, kidneys, liver and the pancreas are toned up.
- Improves the appetite, straightens the chest.

17. Shalabhasana

Method: Lie face down, forehead touching the ground. Keep hands by the side of the body, stretched, heels and soles aligned. Sliding both your hands below the body, place your fists under the groin. Rest your chin on the ground and breathing slowly in, raise both your legs up. It can be started by one leg, then the other leg and both legs. Come back in Shithilasana.

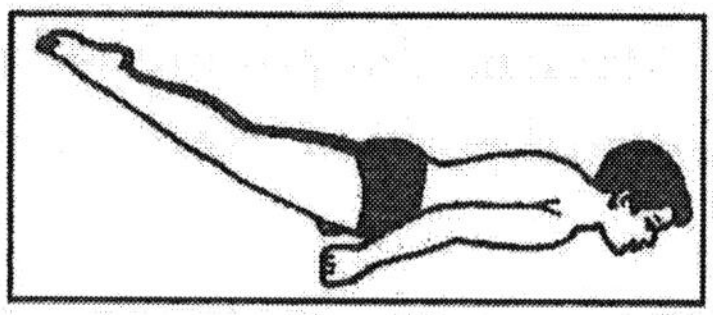

Fig. 17

Benefits:

- It lessens problems of the womb, menstruation and vaginal discharge.
- Low backache, leg pains are eliminated.
- Laziness is washed out. Virility improves.
- It relieves hip-pain and strengthens the heart.
- Lower spine becomes elastic.

18. Mayurasana

Method: Kneel and sit erect on the heels on vajrasana. Open hands together and place the palms on the ground in between the knees with the fingers facing the toes. Place the elbows on the navel area and stretch the legs backward one-by-one and balance carefully. Try bend body forward and the legs will automatically be lifted. Keep the body parallel to the ground and try to raise your head slightly. Balance in this posture for a while and then come to the original position. Rest in shithilasana like child.

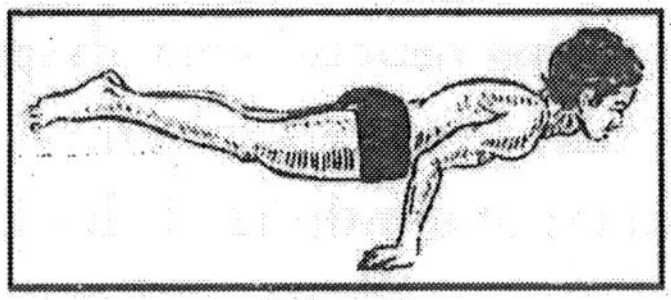

Fig. 18

Benefits:

- Digestive complaints fade away.
- It injects new energy into the systems.
- Regular performance of this asana keeps the old age at bay.
- Prevents-Jaundice, constipation, piles, diabetes etc.
- It removes pot-belly and excess fat.
- Wrists and fore-arms-muscles are strengthened.
- It digests poison if taken.

19. Sheershasana

Method: Sit on the heels touching the knees to the ground. Join hands and interlock the fingers. Place fore-arms on the ground, bending the body forward. Bend further and place the top of head on the pad of cloth. Let the fingers be touching the back portion of the head. Now raise the hip and waist to make a triangle and then slowly bring the feet towards the sky.

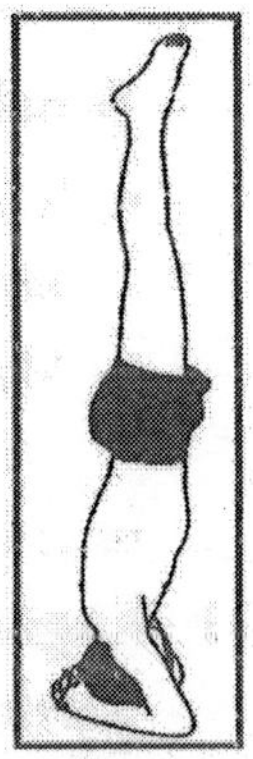

Fig. 19

Gradually raise the legs, thighs, hips waist and back in a straight line. Stand on the head for a while and then slowly come down and stand for a while, then relax.

Benefits:

- Ailments of head, eyes and the ears are cured.
- Excites endocrine glands and regulates their functions.
- Increases memory-power, improves overall development of body and personality.

- It is useful in curing neurasthenia, dyspepsia, constipation, congested throat, liver and spleen, visceroptosis, hernia, seminal weakness and asthma of the nervous and hepatic types.

20. Makarasana: (on Belly)

Method: Lie prone, widen the feet heels inwards touching the ground, fingers outwards. Bending the right hand, place the right palm on the left shoulder. Keeping the left palm on the right shoulder, the chin in front of the hands such that the neck is supported at the point where the two arms cross. Rest and relax.

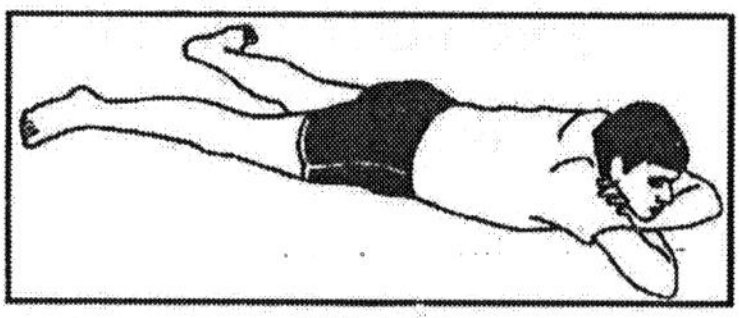

Fig. 20

Benefits:

- It is good for insomnia, high blood pressure, nervousness and indigestion.
- Massage is given to the abdominal organs.
- It is a relaxing asana and eradicates the fatigue.
- It is useful to those whose spine/back is injured.

21. Kagasana

Method: Sit down on your feet. Keep your feet and knees apart. Place your hands on your knees, keep your back erect and look straight ahead. Stay in the position as long as you can.

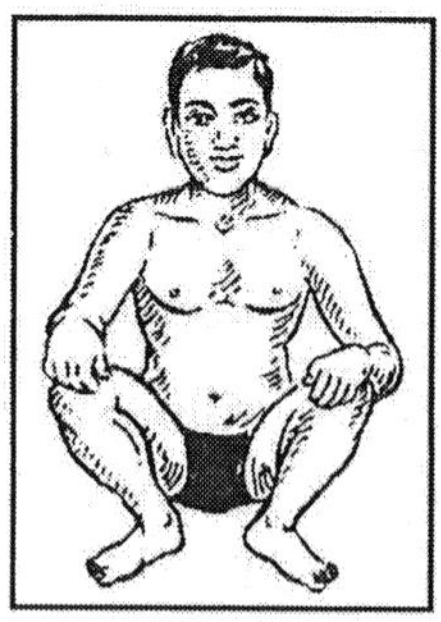

Fig. 21

This asana is also done in slightly different sitting posture (mudra). In that case we keep the feet about ten inches apart. The knees are also kept apart accordingly.

Benefits:

- Practising this asana increases blood circulation to the knees, the thighs, the calves, the hips, the throat etc.
- It increases agility.
- It is used in performing the Kunjal Kriya, Neti Kriya and normal sitting.
- It is natural pose for clearing the bowels.

22. Trikonasana

Method: Stand upright with your legs wide apart. Keeping the right hand up and erect, left hand with the left leg. Bend your body (Trunk) to your left side as much as possible without moving your feet. Right hand will be parallel to the ground. Stay in this position as long as you can. Regain your former position and repeat the process by bending in right side after changing the position of the hands.

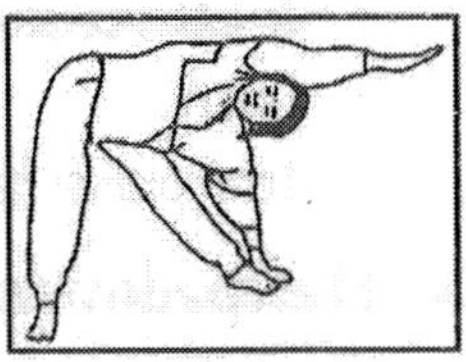

Fig. 22

Benefits:

- Reduces obesity, cures boils, abscesses, backache in the ribs.
- It increases height,
- It removes the weakness of the lungs, sciatica pain etc.

Note: Pregnant women (upto 7 months) should do this asana very slowly.

23. Gomukhasana

Method: Sit down. Bend the left leg at the knee and place the heel on the right side under the anus. Bring the right knee over the left knee and the right heel as close to the left buttock as possible.

Take the right arm behind the back from above and left arm from below so that fingers of both the

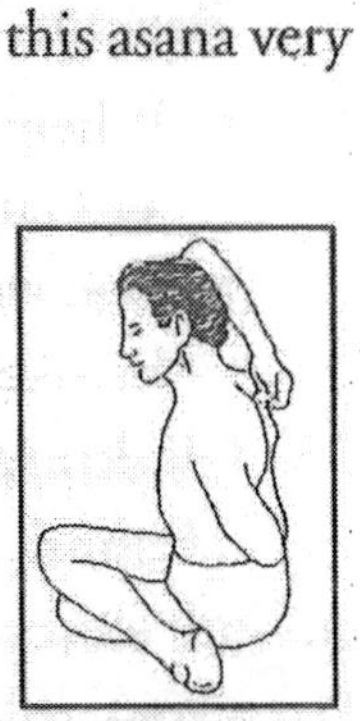

Fig. 23

hands are interlocked behind the back. Normalise the breath. Keep the neck erect. Stay in this position for sometime. Repeat this process on the other side also. When completed take rest.

Benefits:

- Cures seminal weakness, leucorrhea, diabetes, kidney disorder, backpain, neck pain, weakness of the hand nerves, asthma.
- Helps tone up our nervous system and stabilise our mind.
- Unnecessary enlargement of the testicles is prevented.
- It also cures the ailments of thighs, the pelvic, throat and heart.
- It expands the chest and increases the lungs capacity.

24. Hastpadottanasana

Method: Lie down on the ground on your back keeping your legs together and the palms pressed against the outer sides of the thighs. Raise your head, the shoulders, the back and the legs up slowly at the same time. The head and the feet should be raised about one foot above the ground. Maintain this position as long as you can and then slowly regain the former position. Relax.

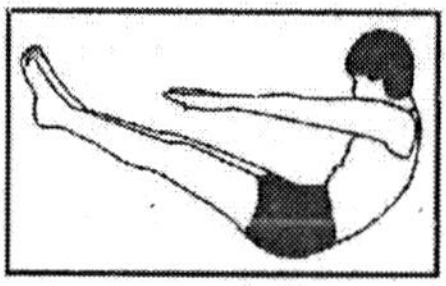

Fig. 24

Benefits:

- It helps to keep the navel in its proper place and prevents and cures ailments of the navel.
- The wind, obesity and diabetes are cured.
- Invokes a balance of mind.

25. Chakrasana

Method: Lie down on your back placing your feet on the ground, close to the buttocks so that your knees point be upwards. Place your palms on the ground on both sides of your head-the elbows pointing towards the sky. Now, supporting yourself on your hands and feet, raise the body up slowly to form an arch. With only the palms and the toes remaining in touch with the ground, stretch your body up as much as possible. Stay in this position as long as you can and then come down slowly to the starting position. Relax.

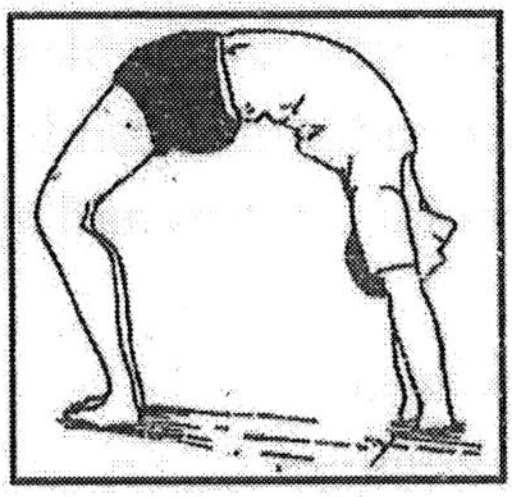

Fig. 25

Benefits:

- The asana strengthens the hands, the arms, the legs, the knees, the waist, the back, the chest and the shoulders.
- It makes the backbone supple, reduces the waist, broadens the chest, the body beautiful.
- Helps to prevent and cure diabetes and obesity.
- Special benefit is setting the displaced navel.
- It is very good for blood circulation and strong nervous system.

26. Ustrasana

Method: Assume sitting posture as in kneeling. Support the body on the toes and the knees and gradually lean backward. Fix the arms from behind and initially put them on heels. Fingers pointing outward and the thumbs towards the toes. Keep the arms straight, slowly lift the

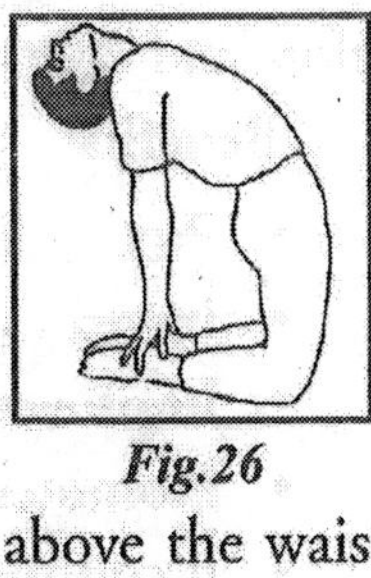

Fig.26

pelvis while taking in the breath, press the body above the waist slowly both outward and upward, throwing the neck downward. Return to kneeling position with exhalation. Sit in vajrasana. Relax.

Benefits:

- Prevents flabbiness and relieves vertebral pressure.
- Promotes spinal circulation. strengthens urogenital muscles.
- Exercises all the deep muscles of the inner side of the thighs, trunk and the neck.
- Sets the slipdisc. Exercise favourable influence on the ovaries, thyroid and other endocrine glands.
- Reduces the extra fat on hips and abdomen. Increases the height.
- It strengthens the heart.

27. Vipreetakarani

Method: Lie down on the ground. Put your palms on the both sides downward. Raise both your legs and hold them at a 30 degree angle without bending at the knees. Increase the angle to 60 degrees and then slowly 90 degrees. Now bend the legs towards your head, and raise your buttocks with both the hands bringing the elbows and the legs in a vertical line. Support the waist with palms. Stay as you can . Slowly remove the support and get the buttocks down. Lower the legs by stages like before and take rest in Shavasana.

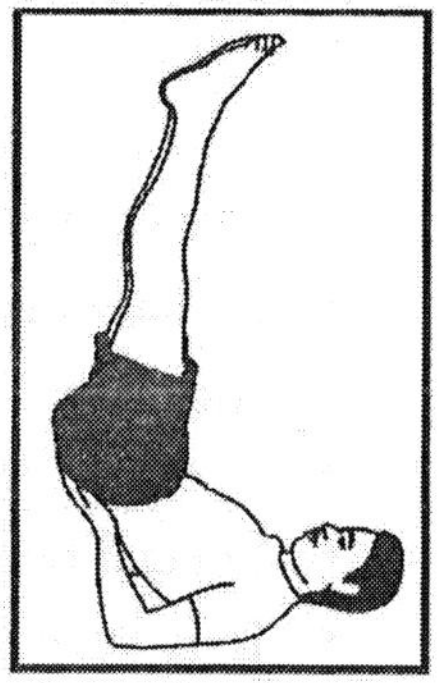

Fig. 27

Benefits:

- Process aids digestion.
- Increases supply of blood to the thorax and the head.
- Improves the blood circulation and cures the varicose veins.
- Promotes health of the sex organs.
- It controls increased blood pressure, pulse and respiration.
- It is good for cerebral anemia, sexual debility, prolapsus of the uterus and congestion etc.

28. Uttanpadasana (Padottanasana)

Method: Lie on spine with your hands on the sides and the feet together. Inhale and hold the breath, then slowly raise both the legs without bending the knees and stop at 30 degree angle. Extend the angle to 60 degrees and then further to 90 degrees. Stay as you can. Return slowly and exhale the breath. Rest a bit.

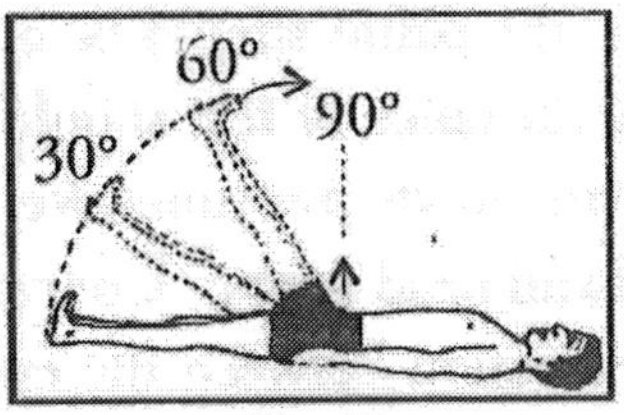

Fig. 28

Benefits:

- The muscles and the organs of the abdominal region are toned up. It removes the constipation.
- The lumber region gets a steady pull and consequently the hip joints become flexible.
- It reduces the fat in the body.

Note: You can perform this asana with one-by-one leg first and with both legs afterwards.

29. Parvatasana

Method: Sit in padmasana. Raise your hands sideward and join them over the head at the same time inhaling. Inhale further and stretch your hands as high as possible. While maintaining the position take normal breathing. While exhaling lower the hands sidewise. Rest.

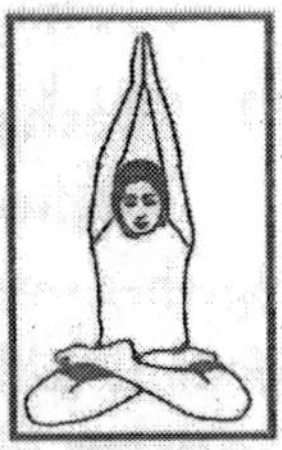

Fig. 29

Benefits:

- Neck and back, abdominal and pelvic muscles are strengthened.

- Keeps the arthritis of the shoulders away.
- Ribs become more flexible.
- It relieves the tension in the neck and shoulders. Loosen the hips.
- Reduces the fatty and flabby abdomen.

30. Shavasana

Method: Lie flat, the palms should be apart from the thighs about 15 degrees. The distance of feet should be about one foot. Inhale deeply and exhale slowly five times. Relax the parts one-by-one from toes to head and head to toes. Concentrate on the breath and focus your concentration between the eyebrows. Do it for 5 minutes.

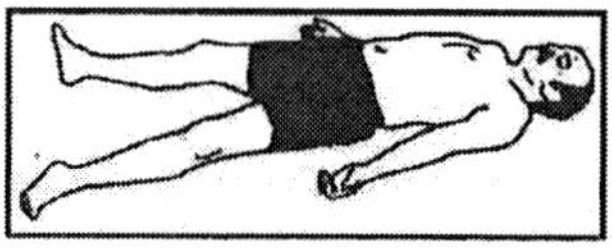

Fig. 30

Benefits:

- Body, mind and heart are relaxed.
- Removes psychosomatic disorders.
- Induces good sleep.
- Reduces B.P. and calms the mind,
- Gives complete rest to all parts of the body.

31. Shashankasana

Method: Sit in vajrasana. Keep the body erect. Raise the arms together over the head. Inhale and stretch the body upward. Bend forward without raising the buttock along with exhaling slowly. Put palms, elbows and forehead on the ground. Relax, inhale, stretch the arms and come back.

Benefits:

- The spine gets complete rest.

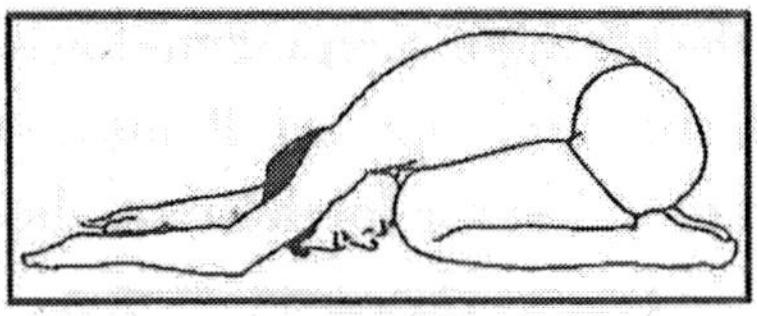

Fig. 31

- Liver, spleen and stomach become activated.
- Breath becomes normal of asthmatic patient.
- It controls the anger and emotions.
- It makes one constructive minded and polite nature.

32. Nuakasana

Method: Lie down on the abdomen. Stretch the hands beyond the head. Inhaling, raise the legs, keeping the heels and toes together at the back and raise the hands in the front. Balance the body at the navel. Now start rolling forward and backward. During the entire process of the asana the feet and arms should remain fully stretched. While exhaling return to the original position and relax.

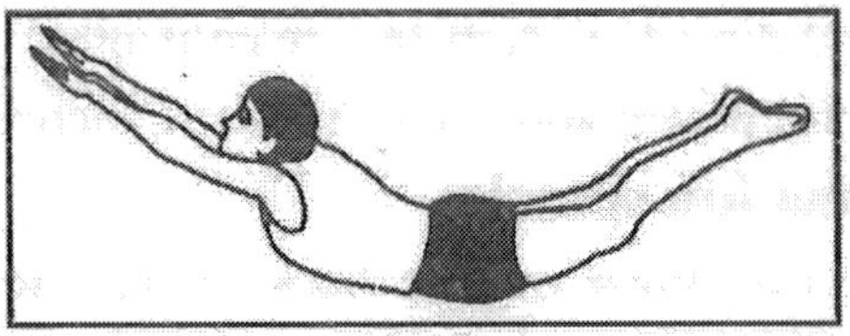

Fig. 32

Benefits:

- Massaging the internal organs of the stomach.
- It controls the obesity, tones up the pancreas gland, helps in proper functioning of liver.
- Makes the digestive system good.
- Curing the indigestion due to overeating, pain in upper part of the navel and abdominal disorders.

33. Janusirasana

Method: Sit on the asana with the legs stretched forward. Bend the left leg and left heel must press perineal space. The sole of the foot should touch the left thigh. Keeping the lower part erect, inhaling the breath, stretch the hands upward. Bend for while exhaling and catch hold the left foot. Put the forehead on the knee.

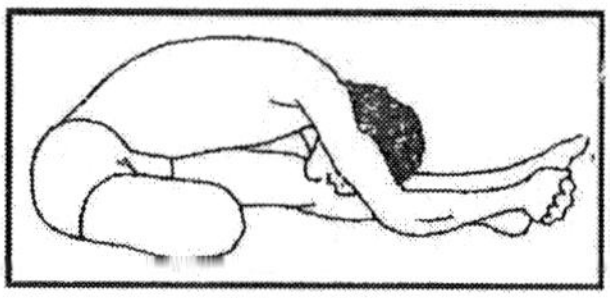

Fig. 33

Rest for a while, normalise the breath. Repeat this practice with the other foot also. Relax.

Benefits:

- Setting right the pelvic region disorders, reproductive cells gastic troubles, obstruction of urine, and heat of the intestines.
- It cures the sciatica nerve pain and spine becomes flexible.
- It strengthens the legs.
- Seminal disorders, diabetes are controlled.
- Digestive power and pran shakti are increased.

34. Makrasana (on spine)

Method: Lie down on the back. Keep the heels and toes together. Fold the legs in such a manner that the heels should touch the hips. Spread the arms to the right and left sides in a line. Palms up. Inhale and move the knees to the left and neck towards the right, place the right ear and the knees on the ground. Returnback with exhaling. Repeat this process to the other side and Relax.

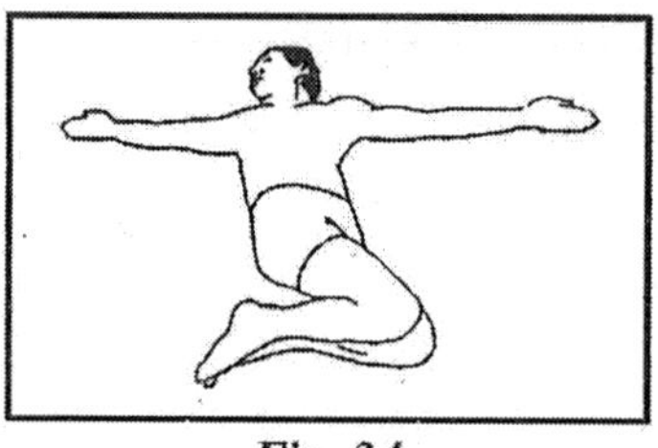

Fig. 34

Benefits:

- Spine becomes elastic, ribs and lungs become strong.
- Relief in breathing problems and cures diabetes.
- It removes the constipation, obesity, spinal disorders as cervical, slipdisc and backache.
- It normalises the blood pressure.

35. Greeva Chakrasana

Method: Sit in any meditative pose. Turn your neck right, left, front and back slowly three-four times. Move the neck in a circle clockwise and anti-clockwise four times.

Benefits:

- B.P. remains in control.
- E.N.T. regional nerves become strong.
- Eyesight increases.
- No possibility of cervical.

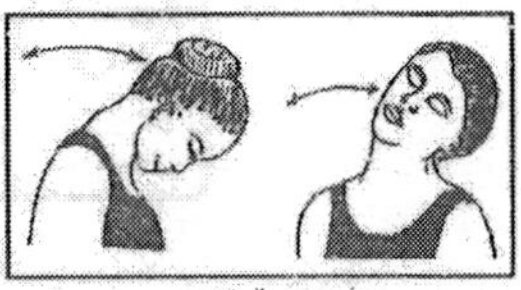

Fig. 35

36. Shithilasana

Method: Lie flat on the abdominal at full length. Resting the right ear on the ground. Fold the left foot at 90 degrees. Bring the left heel to the right knee. Left hand palm may be placed in front of the face, shoulders are relaxed. Normal breathing with closed eyes. Repeat the same process on the other side.

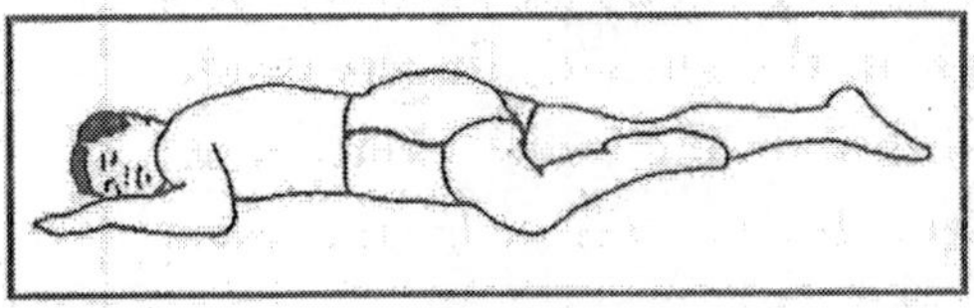

Fig. 36

Benefits:

- It gives complete relief from fatigue.
- Helps in sleeping, sets right the B.P. as Shithilasana on right side lowers the H.B.P., fever and headache, on the left side.

- Shithalasana increases the body temperature and the cold removed.

37. Sarpasana

Method: Lie down on the abdomen. Place the hands on the back with fingers interlocked. Stretch the heels and toes together without bending the knees and inhaling raise the body from the front and the rear. Now start rolling on the ground right and left side of the body as long as breath is inside. If need of taking a breath is felt take on either side. Return slowly to the first position and rest in shithilasana.

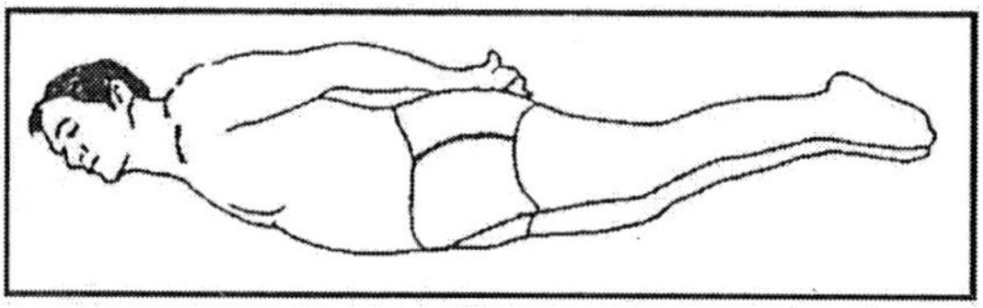

Fig. 37

Benefits:

- All the organs of the abdomen are nicely massaged.
- It relieves constipation and increases appetite.
- Chest expands and shoulders become strong. Abdomen and the body become supple and well.

38. Sinhasana

Method: Sit in padmasana, move forward, put the palms on the ground, fingers inside. Open the mouth and tongue out. Concentrate on the Nasagra. Inhale and make the sweet voice 5 times and return.

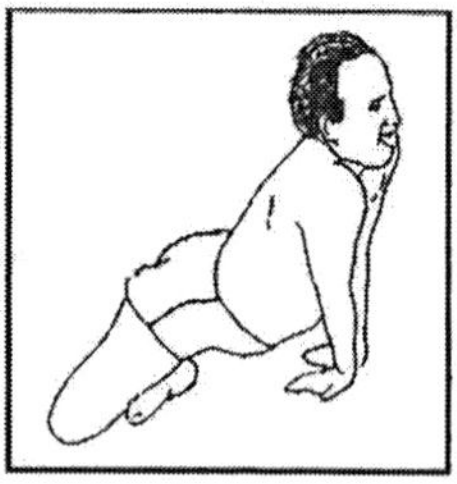

Fig. 38

Benefits:

- Removes the throat ailments like tonsils, lungs and seminal glands. It keeps the food pipe clean.
- Three bandhas capacity increases.

- It promotes the healthiness of eyes, ears and nose.

39. Kamar Chakrasana

Method: Sit on the asana. Spread your feet on the either side as wide as possible. Hold the left toe with the right hand, and the left hand take in back side. Touch the nose to the left knee. Inhale and change the other side. Repeat it 5 to 10 times slowly. Exhale when you bend. Relax.

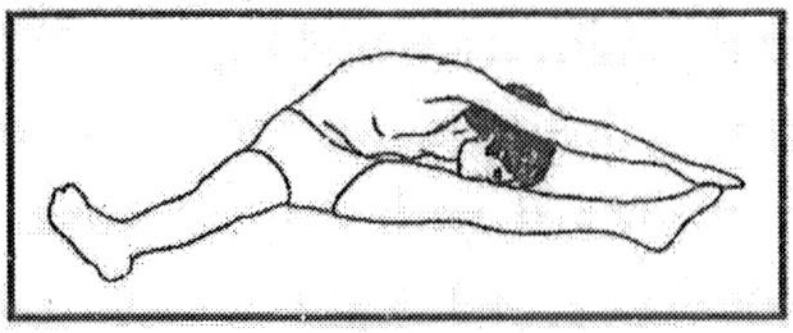

Fig. 39

Benefits:

- It makes the spine flexible, the sciatica nerve pain removed, lower portion of the waist becomes flexible.
- Forward bending becomes easy.
- The body becomes supple.

40. Ardha Chakrasana (Satubandhasana Kandharasana)

Method: Lie on the spine. Bend both the knees. Catch the ankles with respective hands. Inhale and raise the abdomen up. Stay a while. Exhale and come back. Take rest.

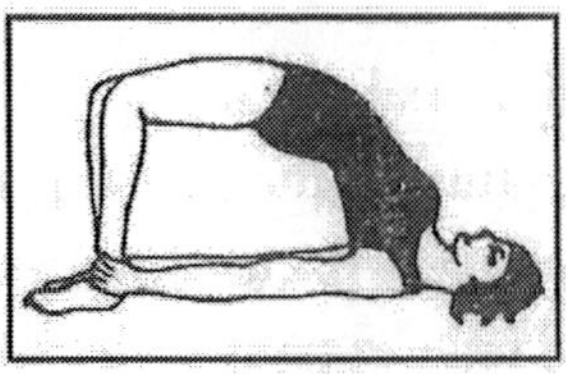

Fig. 40

Benefits:

- It cures indigestion and gas troubles.
- Makes the spine flexible.
- Shoulders, arms, legs, neck are strengthened.

- It cures bronchial and Thyroid disorders.
- It keeps the navel in its position. It removes stomach pain, backache, infertility, bleeding and uterus, menstrual, and woman related disorders.

41. Expadothanasana

Method: Lie on the back. Keep the heels together. Put the hands on the floor by the sides of the body. Stretch the feet forward. Inhale slowly. Lift the right stretched leg up at 90 degrees. Hold the breath and remain in this position for 5-8 seconds. Take rest for 6-8 seconds and practise it with the other leg. Repeat only four times in the beginning by each leg. Increase its practice gradually.

Note: To get more benefit keep the heel 2" up of one leg and the other leg should be at 90°.

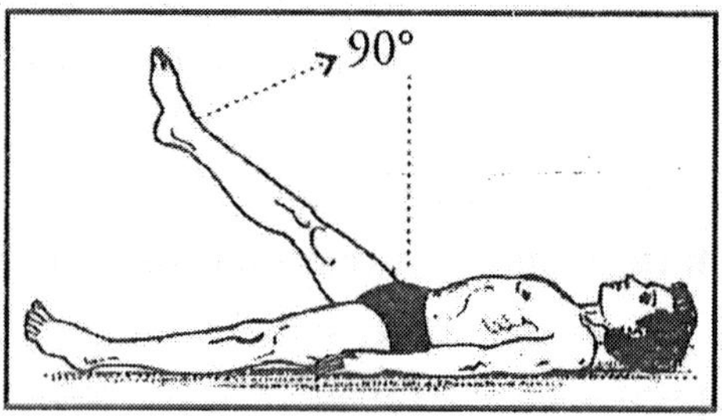

Fig. 41

Benefits:

- It reduces abdominal obesity.
- It relieves pain during menstrual periods.
- It removes swelling in the legs, tones up the blood circulation in the legs and relieves pain in the knees and the lower parts of the legs.
- It relieves stomach pain and tones up the liver, the spleen and the kidneys.
- It cures indigestion, gas-trouble and intestinal disorders. It strengthens the intestines.

- It has a good effect on the upper part of the body (Thorax). It strengthens the lungs and spine.
- It has a good effect in conditioning the mind.
- It tones up the muscles of the sex glands and enhances potency.

42. Natarajasana

Nataraja means Lord Shiva. Natrajasnas means Lord Shivas pose in his cosmic dance mudra.

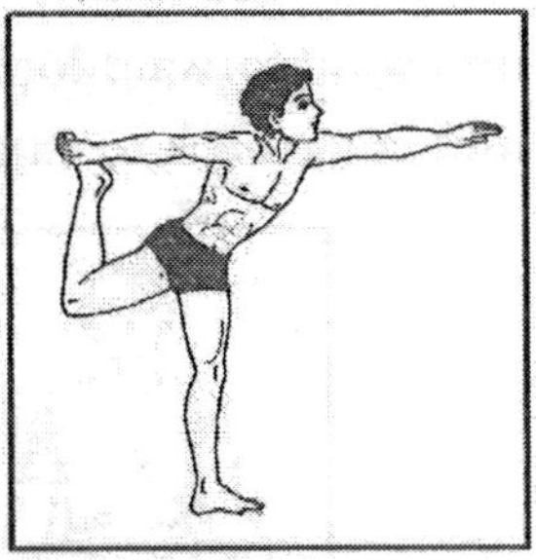

Fig. 42

Method: Stand erect with the legs straight. Keep the arms straight by the sides and look straight. Bend either leg at the knee and raise it backwards. Hold the foot with the corresponding hand. Stretch the other arm in the opposite direction and look straight in that direction. Hold the position for 10 seconds. Repeat the exercise standing on the other leg. In the beginning this asana can be practised four times a day. Later, it can be practised six times a day. Normal breathing during practice.

Benefits:

- It relieves the pain in the waist and makes the waist flexible. It brings the flexibility to the spine.
- This asana balances the nervous system.
- It develops control of the body and mental concentration. It keeps the calm state of mind.
- It makes the legs supple.
- Activates the rudra granthi and the Agya Chakra by Channelising the flow of pran to them.
- It expands the chest cavity and relieves bronchial spasms.
- Strengthens the lower limbs as it bears the weight of the body one-by-one.

- The asana is good for curing indigestion, chronic fever, dysentery, heart-disease, T.B., asthma, diabetes etc.
- This asana is useful for the cure of stiffness in the joints of the lumber region.
- This asana helps the mind to be firm, attentive and alert.
- It is helpful to control the seminal energy, vritis and pran.
- Siddhasana increases power of concentration.
- It supplies sufficient blood to the pelvic region, cures syphilis, gonorrhoea, arthritis and keeps the body in poise and equilibrium.
- This asana is beneficial for all sportsmen and women.

46. Padahastasana

It is a pose where the hands (Hasta) are brought closer the feet (Pada). This asana is for beginners.

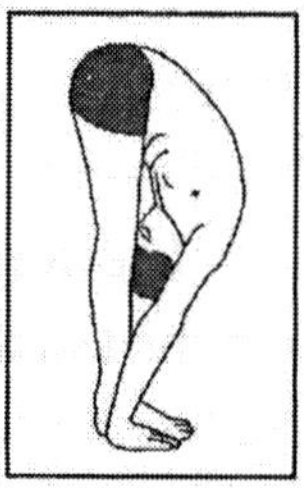

Fig. 46

Method: Stand upright feet together. Breathe in deeply. Raise the hands high over the head, palms forward. The upper arms covering the ears, exhale and keep the legs locked. Bend forward from the waist. Put the palms near the foot each side or catch the ankles. Touch the forehead from knees. Stay a bit and comeback with stretched hands slowly.

Benefits:

- It removes obesity.
- It tones up the nervous system.
- Massages the abdominal organs.
- It is excellent for loosening the shoulders and upper back, limbering the spine and toning the arms, legs and hips.
- It also feeds the facial tissues and scalp with blood and improves the circulation.

- It cures the disease of the toes, invigorates the weak, abdominal diseases, strengthens the chest. Body becomes handsome and radiant.
- Makes the body light, flexible, blood supply to the brain to remove fatigue due to brain work.
- It cures sciatica, constipation, dislocated navel (dharan) and obesity (motapa).

47. Vakrasana

Method: Sit on the asana with the legs stretched out. Place the left leg near the right knee, stretching out the left hand behind the back, with the palm of the hand flat resting on the ground. Then press the left knee with the right arm and put palm on the ground. Keep the waist erect and look as far as possible backward. Practice this asana on the other side. Repeat it 4-6 times a day turning to the left side and to the right side alternately. Gradually, increase the time, the limit five minutes.

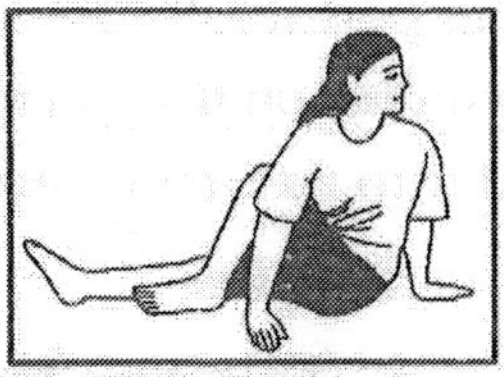

Fig. 47

Benefits:

- This asana invigorates the muscles of the loins (lower back)
- The mouth of the Shushumna opens and Kundalini shakti is sublimated.
- This asana strengthens the spine and activates the nerves.
- This reduces the fat from the waist.
- It is beneficial for the liver, spleen and pancreas.
- It cures stomach disorders and strengthens the intestines.

Variation: The foot can be put beyond the knee and may be caught knee by hand.

48. Vrikshasana

'Vriksha' means a tree. In this asana the body assumes the shape of a tree. So it is called Vrikshasana.

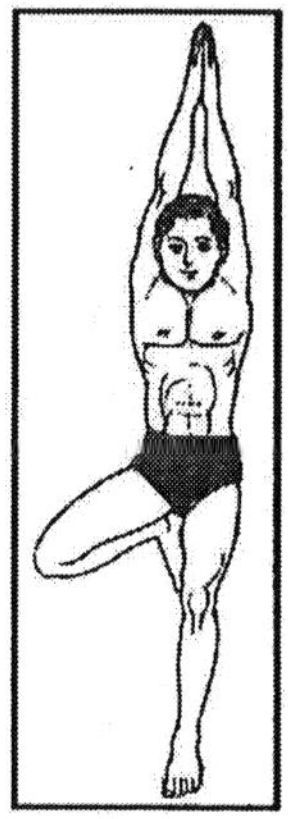

Fig. 48

Method: Stand on either leg. If difficulty is experienced to balance the body on one leg, take the support of a wall. Bend the other leg at the knee and place its heel at the root of the thigh of the former leg as shown in the figure. Join the palms and raise the arms. Straight over the head. Inhale slowly. Hold this position for about 10 seconds. Repeat the pose, standing on the other leg. The exercise can be practise four to six times a day.

Benefits:

- This asana tones up all the joints of the body.
- It supplies blood to the blood vessels of the toes, the knees, the elbows, etc., in sufficient quantity.
- The hands and the legs become flexible by the practice of this asana.
- It makes the chest shapely.
- It has the effect of mild traction on the spine.
- It is useful for nervousness, debility, pain and ache in the chest and sides.
- It is helpful increasing the height of young children and adolescents.
- It develops the balance of mind, concentration and tolerance power.

49. Padangusthasana

Method: Keep the left heel in between the genitals and the rectum. Keep the right leg above the left thigh. Now rest both the hands on both sides, balance the body on the ankle. Lift the hands

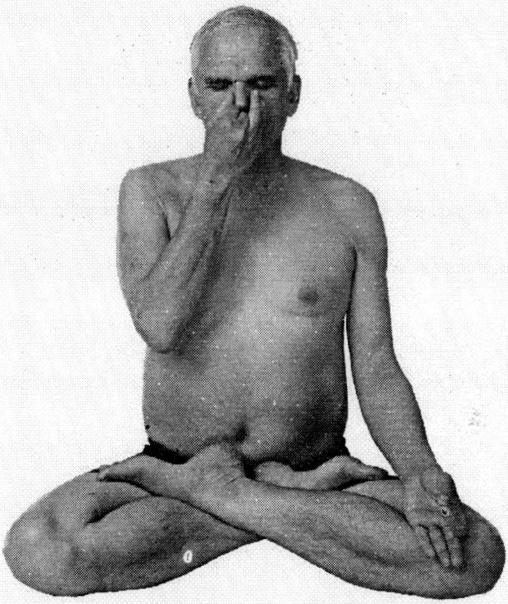

NADI SHODHAN PRANAYAMA

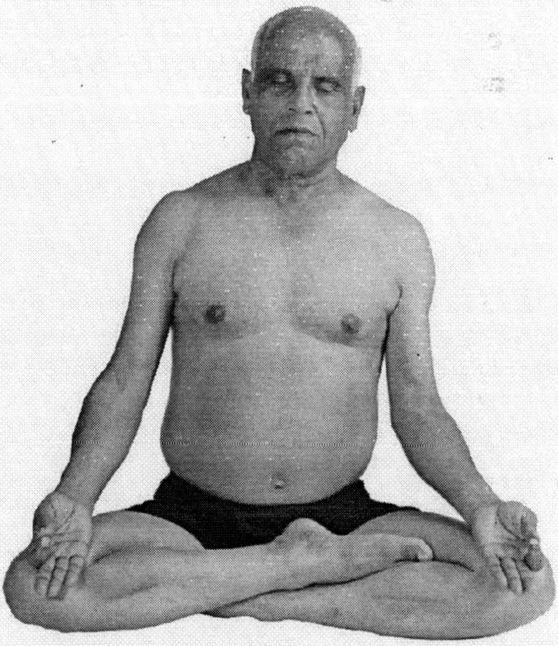

SIDDHASANA

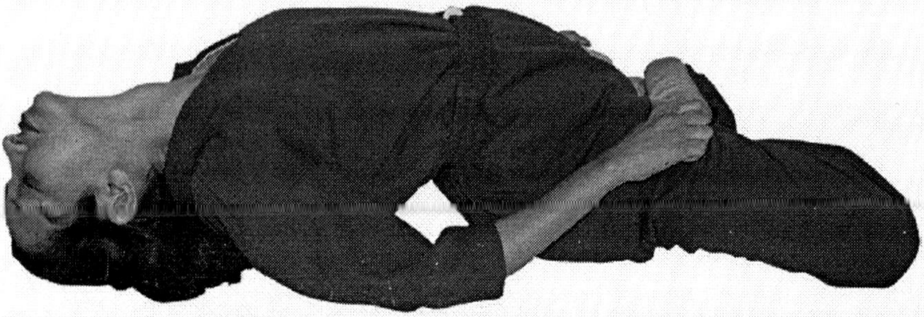

MATSYASANA

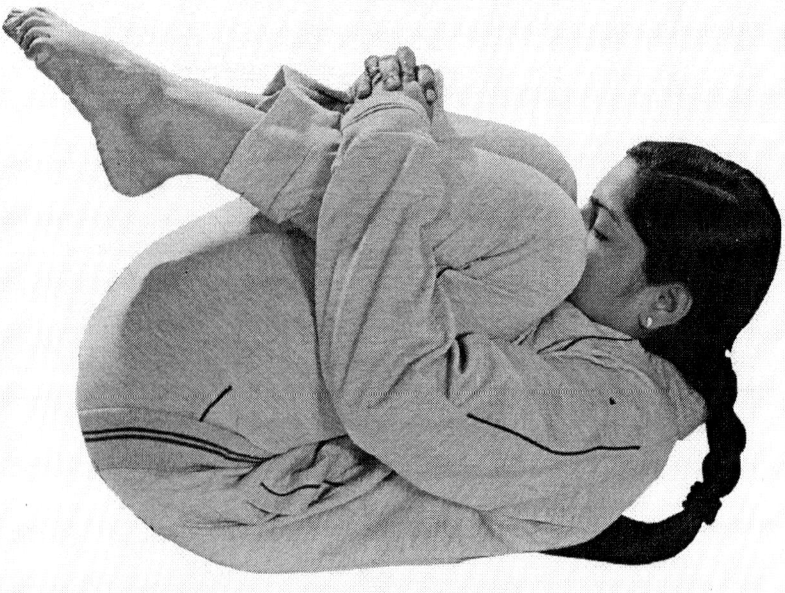

PAWANA MUKTASANA

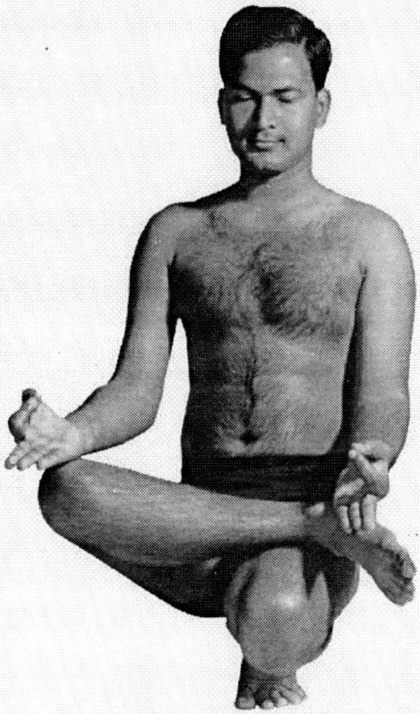
PADANGUSTHASANA

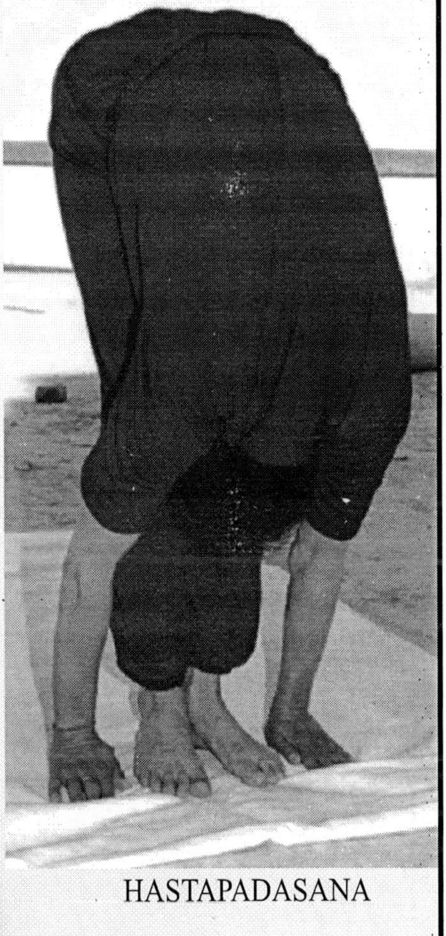
HASTAPADASANA

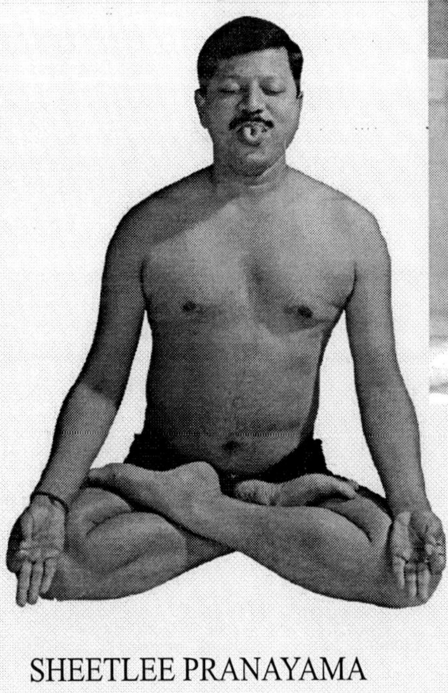
SHEETLEE PRANAYAMA

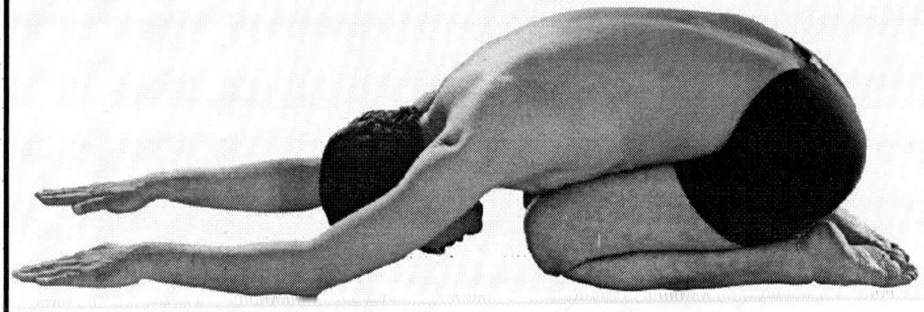

SHASHANKASANA

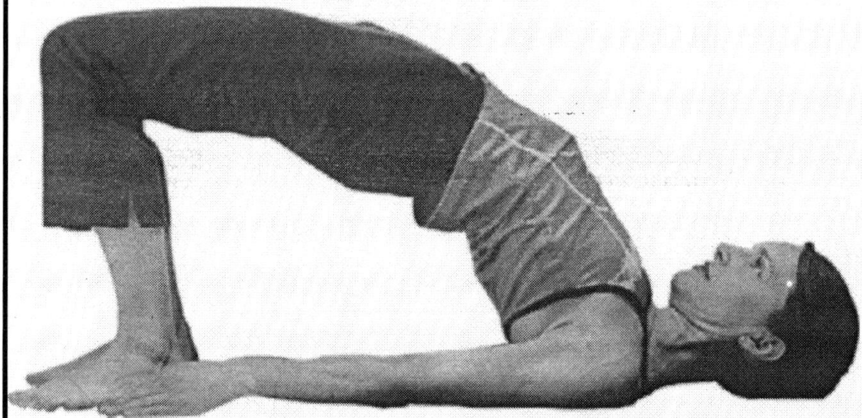

SETUBANDASANA

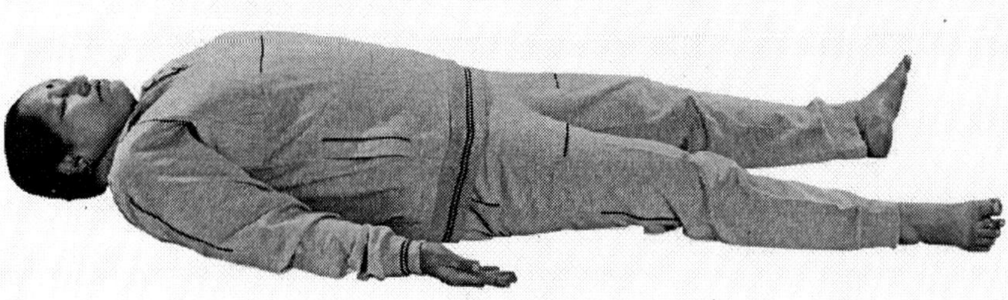

SHAVASANA

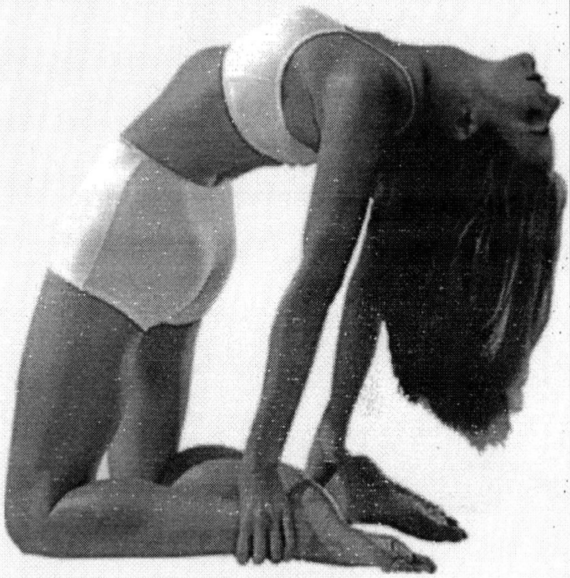

USTRASANA

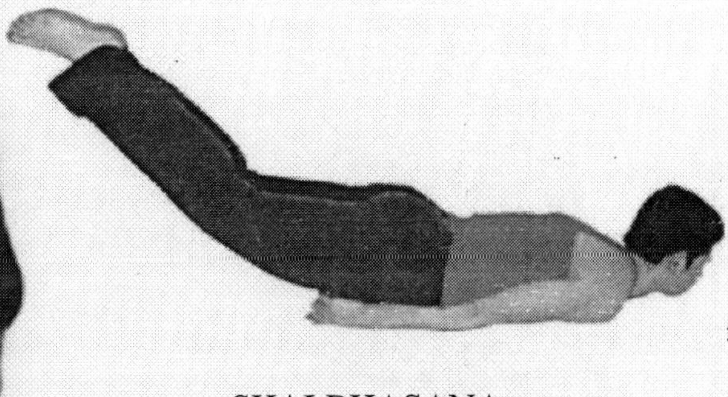

SHALBHASANA

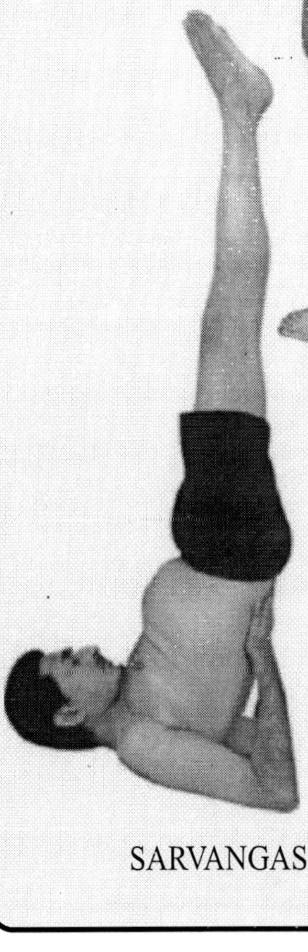

SARVANGASANA

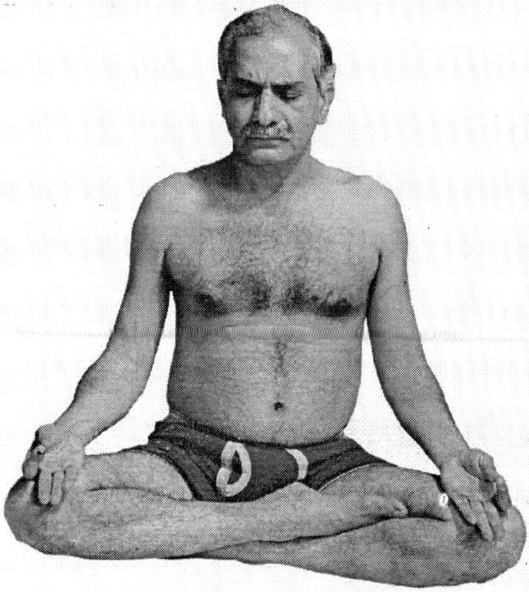

SWASTIKASANA

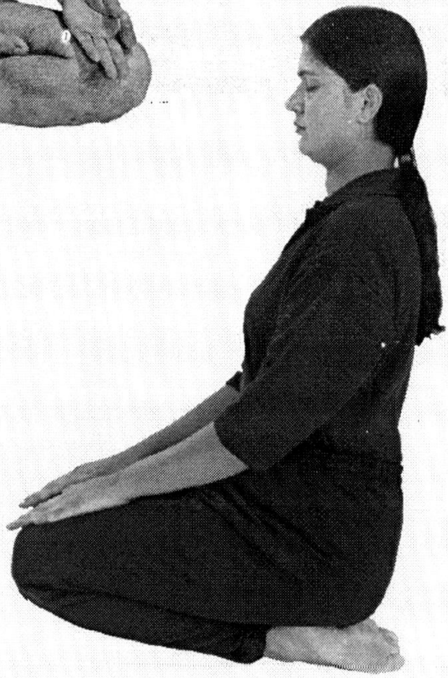

VAJRASANA

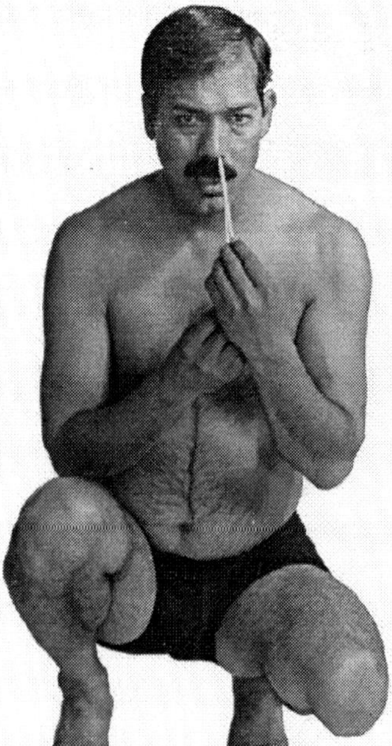

SUTRA NETI

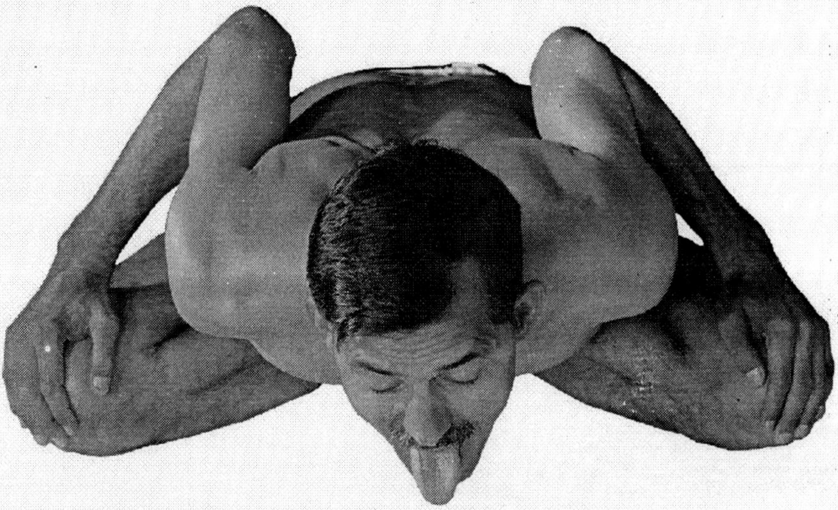

PLAVANI PRANAYAMA

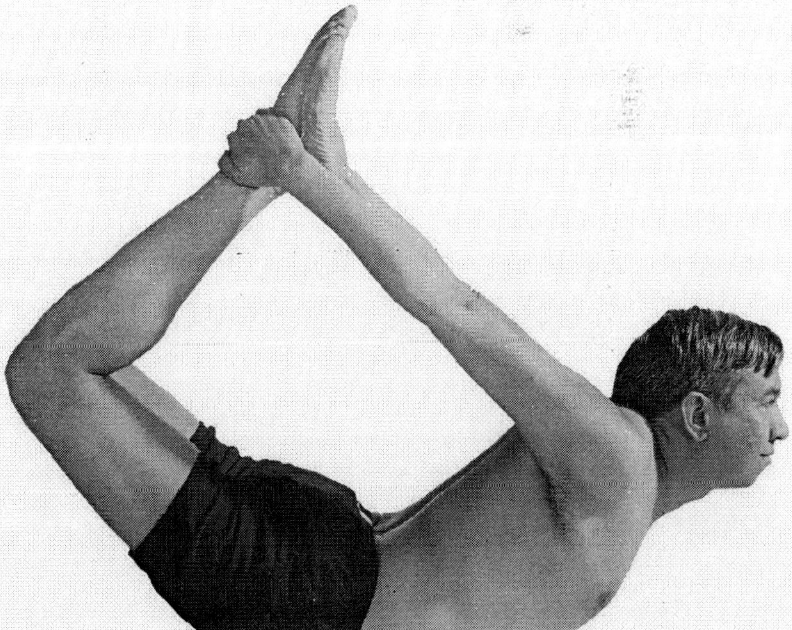

DHANURASANA

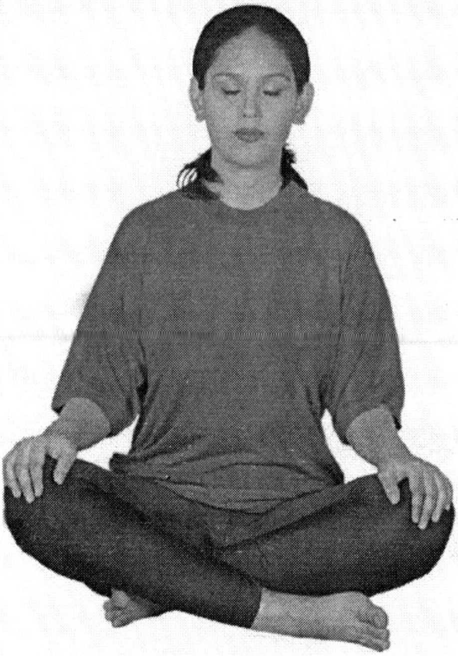

SUKHASANA

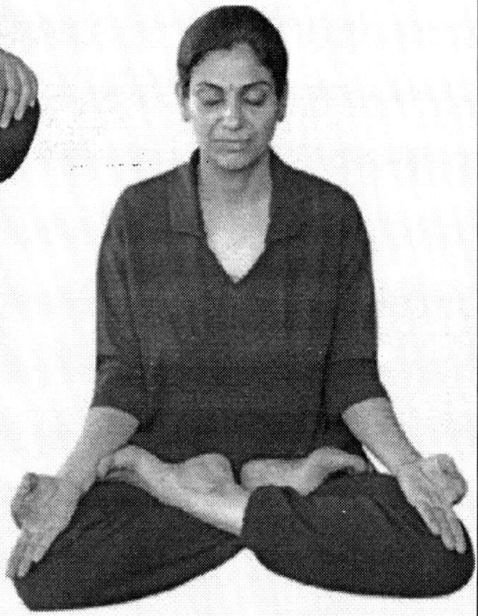

PADMASANA

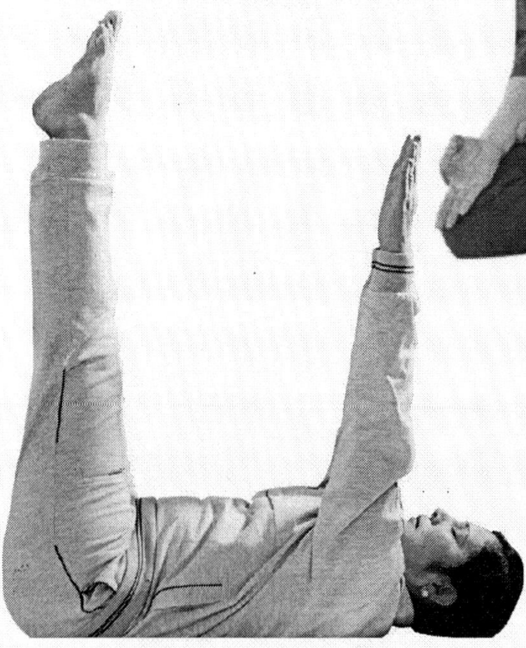

PADOTTANASANA

as namaskara position. Gaze on a fixed point ahead. Remain in this position for sometimes. Keep the breathing normal. After doing with one leg repeat the asana with other leg.

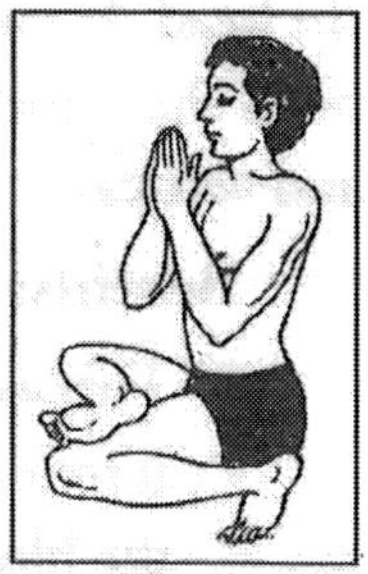

Fig. 49

Benefits:

- It increases the strength, intelligence and vigour.
- It is useful for celibacy
- When practised for long time, Kundalini awakes and the sperm rises above.
- It regulates the reproductive system.
- It prevents spermatorrhea.
- It also remedies flat feet and strengthens the toes and ankles.
- The falling tendency of the semen is stopped.
- Eye sight remains intact due to its impact on our toes and feet.
- It helps balanced development of the body and self-control.
- Nerves and veins of the feet become strong and elastic.

50. Marjariasana (Catspose)

This is a simplest and energy blocking asana.

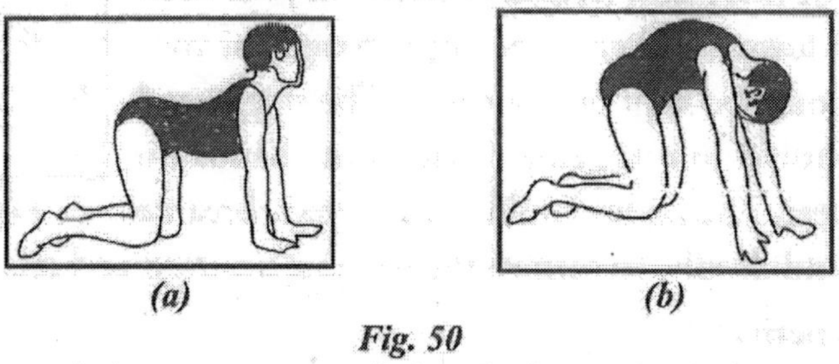

(a) *(b)*

Fig. 50

Method: Sit in vajrasana. Raise the buttocks and stand on the knees and at the same time, place both hands flat on the floor in front of the body. Keep head under the shoulders. Inhale and raise the head. Then exhale and lower the head and arch the spine. Again, bend the spine and raise the head. The arms are to be kept straight and vertical.

Benefits:

- This asana is extremely beneficial for pregnant women.
- It tones up the nervous system, adrenal glands and normalise the blood circulation.
- It strengthens the muscles of the arms, legs and makes the waist supple.
- It can also cure asthma and kidney-ailments.
- This asana also feels good if you have a gastric problem and you are wanting to relieve yourself.
- It relaxes the back, back pain and hips/legs/pains.

Precaution:

1. If you have high blood pressure, stay in the both positions but avoid getting the head down.

51. Utkatasana

It is another powerful and popular asana.

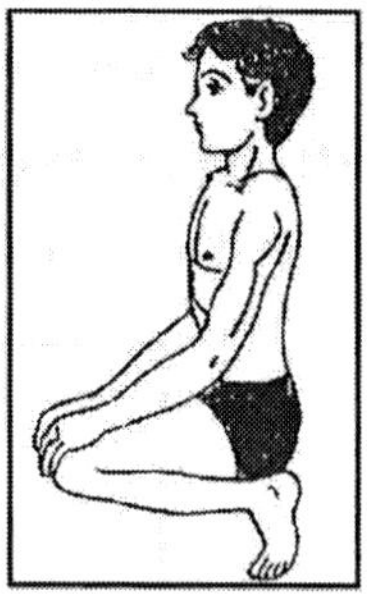

Fig. 51

Method: Stand on your toes and raise the heels as high as you can. Keep the palms on the waist. Lower the body slow by and sit down on your heels without lowering them. The entire weight of your body should be kept on your toes. The thighs and calves should join together. Place your hands on your knees. The body should remain erect, breathe slowly and deeply. Return to the original position and relax.

Benefits:

- This asana strengthens all the muscles of the body in general and the muscles of toes, ankles, legs and feet in particular.

- It removes impurities in blood.
- It cures sexual disease of women and controls the sexual energies.
- It maintains the equilibrium and balance.
- It can also stimulate nervous system.
- It is extremely beneficial for the football players.
- It is useful for Jalavasti, Pawanvasti for emptying the intestines.
- It helps in developing a correct posture for the spine.
- It is useful in during pregnancy.

Note:

1. Pregnant ladies stand near the wall they can open their knees. Wall will support your back.
2. Do not do this if you have severe painful varicose veins or piles or stitches in your cervix, and bleeding in pregnancy.

Avoid these Asanas if.....

1. **Padmasana:** If you have recently strained or fractured your ankle, if you have a knee problem or if you have varicose veins.
2. **Vajrasana:** If you have a bad ankle or a knee fractured.
3. **Siddhasana:** If you have sciatica or any sacral infections. It is prohibited for ladies for long time.
4. **Tadasana (Standing):** People who are too weak to balance the body on the toes may do this asana lying on the floor.
5. **Trikonasana:** If you have serious respiratory problems, if you are pregnant.
6. **Bhujangasana:** If you have a bratus hernia or a hyperactive thyroid.
7. **Shalbhasana:** If you have high blood pressure or heart trouble.

8. **Dhanurasana:** If you have H.B.P., hernia, duodenal ulcer/ peptic ulcer.
9. **Pawanmuktasana:** If you have cervical spondylitis, do not lift the head. Practice only leg position.
10. **Padhastasana:** If you have a slipped disc or a middle ear disturbance.
11. **Sinhasana:** If you have H.B.P./Heart trouble.
12. **Suptvajrasana:** If you cannot do vajrasana comfortably, if there is any injury in the ankle or knee joint.
13. **Sarvangasana:** If you have any serious medical problem including H.B.P./L.B.P., 1. heart problem, 2. weak eye capillary 3. middle ear trouble, 4. People with slipped disc trouble, spondylitis.
14. **Paschimottanasana:** If you have hernia, an enlarged liver or spleen, H.B.P., Constipation. Do not hold the pose for too long as it may aggravate it instead of curing it.
15. **Halasana:** If you have cervical spondylitis or any pain in the neck.
16. **Parbatasana:** If you have ulscers or any serious lower back problems.
17. **Ushtrasana:** If you have a frail constitution, inadequate stamina and find the asthma strenuous.
18. **Ardhamatsyendrasana:** If you have duodenal or peptic ulcer.
19. **Matsyasana:** If you have either an ear infection or middle ear problem.
20. **Chakrasana:** If you have H.B.P. or coronary complaints, ulcers, hernia or have recently had either a fracture or undergone medical operation.

21. **Shirshasana:** If you have aching or running ears, very weak eyes, H.B.P., Heart, trouble. It must also be avoided by those who do not practice it regularly.
22. **Janushirasana:** If you have ulcers or any serious lower back problem.
23. **Mayurasanas:** If you have H.B.P., hernia, peptic or duodenal ulcers.
24. **Surya Namaskara:** If you have back pain avoid the third and tenth positions.

Yogabhyas Programmes

A. 15 Minutes Programme

S.No.	Posture/Kriya	Time
1.	Uddiyan Bandha (Abdominal Contraction)	1 minute
2.	Sarvangasana (The Shoulder Sland)	1 minute
3.	Halasana (The Plow)	1 minute
4.	Bhujangasana (The Cobra)	1 minute
5.	Paschimottanasana (Posterior Stretch)	1 minute
6.	Dhanurasana (The Bow)	1 minute
7.	Sheersasana (The Headstand)	1 minute
	Take Rest between yogasanas and pranayamas	3 minutes
	Pranayama (Breathing exercise)	
8.	Kapalbhati (The Cleansing Breath)	1 minute
9.	Bhastrika (The Bellows Breath)	1 minute
10.	Ujjai (The Audible Breath)	1 minute
11.	Shavasana (The Corpse Posture)	2 minutes
	Total Time	15 minutes
	Note: Rest Pauses between yogabhyas	

B. Five Minutes Programme

S.No.	Posture/Kriya	Time
1.	Marjari Asana (Cat stretch)	$2\frac{1}{2}$ minutes
2.	• Comfortable Pranayama (Deep breathing) • The Cleansing Breath. (Kapalbhati Pranayama)	$2\frac{1}{2}$ minutes
	Total Time	5 minutes

C. 15 Minutes Programme for Women

S.No.	Posture/Kriya	Time
1.	Sarvangasana (Shoulder Sland)	1.30 Seconds
2.	Bhujangasana (Cobra Pose)	1.30 Seconds
3.	Paschimottanasana (The Posterior Stretch)	1.30 Seconds
4.	Dhanurasana (The Bow)	1.30 Seconds
5.	Parvatasana (The Mountains)	1.30 Seconds
	Breathing Exercise	
6.	Kapalbhati (Cleansing Breath)	1.30 Seconds
7.	Ujjai (Audible Breath)	1.30 Seconds
8.	Shavasana (Corpse Pose)	2.30 Seconds
	Rest Pauses between yogabhyasa	2.00 Seconds
	Total Time	15 Minutes

D. Daily Practice for Women

S.No.	Yogasana	Minimum Duration	Fortnightly increase	Maximum Duration	Remarks
1.	Padmasana	1 minute	1 minute	20 minutes	
2.	Sarvangasana	30 sec.	30 sec.	12 minutes	
3.	Matsyasana	10 sec.	10 sec.	4 minutes /	⅓ of above

4.	Halasana	15 sec.	15 sec.	3 minutes
5.	Bhujangasana	5 sec 3 Rounds	5 sec. 1 Round	20 sec. 6 Rounds
6.	Shalbhasana	—do—	—do—	—do— 6 Rounds
7.	Paschimottana-sana	10 sec.	10 sec.	5 minutes
8.	Parvatasana	15 sec.	10 sec.	4 minutes
9.	Shavasana	10 sec.	5 minutes	1 hour

Note: This programme is recommended for daily practice as soon as puberty sets in.

E. Daily Programme for Women (Middle Age)

S.No.	Yogasana/ Bandha	Maximum Duration	Increase Fortnightly
1.	Padmasana	1-20 minutes	1 minute
2.	Sarvangasana	1-12 minutes	30 seconds
3.	Matsyasana	1-4 minutes	10 seconds
4.	Bhujangasana	5-30 seconds 3-5 turns	5 seconds
5.	Shalbhasana	5-15 seconds	5 seconds
6.	Paschimottanasana	15 sec-3 mts	10 seconds
7.	Ashwini Mudra	15 counts to the minute to -60 counts	5 counts
8.	Parvatasana	30 sec. to 3 mts.	30 seconds
9.	Uddiyan Bandha	5-15 sec., 3-5 turns	5 sec.
10.	Nauli	—do—	—do—
11.	Shavasana	20mts to 1 hour	10 minutes

Note: Uddiyan Bandha and Nauli are strictly forbidden to those girls in whom the periodic function is not fully established. But they are recommended for older girls in whom the function is well established in its regularity but is not otherwise normal.

- Walking for sometime daily for a fortnight or so before adopting this course is strongly recommended. It is common knowledge that an anaemic girl/women needs special care about nutrition.
- This course is also excellent for preparing a girl for marriage in which case Uddiyan and Nauli should be included in it.
- It is good for middle age women.

F. Course for changing women (old)

S.No.	Yogasana/ Bandha	Maximum Duration	Increase Fortnightly
1.	Padmasana	1-20 minutes	by 1 minute
2.	Vipreet Karani/ Sarvangasana	30 sec. -8minutes	30 seconds
3.	Bhujangasana	5-25 seconds 5 Turns	5 seconds
4.	Parvatasana	30 sec.-8 min.	15 seconds
5.	Paschimottanasana	15 sec.-3 min.	10 seconds
6.	Ashwini Mudra	15-16 counts	5 counts
7.	Ardha-Matsyendrasana	30 sec.-3 min.	15 counts
8.	Janushirasana	15 sec.-3 min.	10 counts
9.	Yogamudra	15 sec.-10 min.	20 counts
10.	Shavasana	30 min. each time Morning, Noon, Night	—

G. For Vigorous Young Men (I)

S.No.	Yogasana/ Bandha	Minimum Duration	Maximum Duration	Increase Fortnightly
1.	Sheersasana	1 min.	1 min.	15 min.
2.	Shavasana	20 min.	5 min.	1 hour
	(II)			
3.	Sarvangasana	1 min.	1 min.	12 min.
4.	Matsyasana	20 sec.	20 sec.	4 min.
5.	Halasana	1 min.	30 sec.	3 min.
6.	Bhujangasana	10 sec., 3 Turns	5 sec.	30 sec., 6 Turns
7.	Shalbhasana	5 sec., 3 Turns	3 sec.	15 sec., 6 Turns
8.	Paschimottanasana	15 sec.	10 sec.	3 min.
9.	Parvatasana	15 sec.	15 sec.	4 min.
10.	Aradha Matsyendrasana	1 min.	30 sec.	3 min.
11.	Uddiyan Bandha	3 turns	1 turn	7 turns
12.	Nauli	–do–	–do–	–do–
13.	Shavasana	20 min.	5 min.	1 hour

H. For Weak Young Men (III)

S.No.	Yogasana/ Bandha	Minimum Duration	Fortnightly Increase	Maximum Fortnightly
1.	Sarvangasana	30 Sec.	—	8 min.
2.	Matsyasana	10 Sec.	—	3 min.
3.	Bhujangasana	10 Sec.	5 Sec.	30 Sec.
4.	Shalbhasana	5 Sec.	3 Sec.	15 Sec.
5.	Paschimottanasana	10 Sec.	10 Sec.	3 min.
6.	Parvatasana	10 Sec.,	10 Sec.	1 min.
7.	Yoga Mudra	30 Sec.	30 Sec.	4 min.
8.	Shavasana	20 Sec.	05 min.	1 hour

I. For Middle Aged Men (35-45 yrs.) (IV)

S.No.	Yogasana/ Bandha	Minimum Duration	Fortnightly Increase	Maximum Fortnightly
1.	Sarvangasana	30 sec.	10 sec.	6 min.
2.	Matsyasana	10 sec.	10 sec.	2 min
3.	Bhujangasana	10 sec.	05 sec.	30 sec.
4.	Paschimottanasana	15 sec.	15 sec.	3 min.
5.	Parvatasana	10 sec.	10 sec.	4 min.
6.	Shavasana	25 sec.	5 min.	1.30 min.

J. For Middle Aged Men (46-56 yrs.) (V)

S.No.	Yogasana/ Bandha	Minimum Duration	Fortnightly Increase	Maximum Fortnightly
1.	Padmasana	1 min.	1 min.	10 min.
2.	Parvatasana	10 sec.	10 sec.	4 min.
3.	Paschimottanasana	10 sec.	10 sec.	3 min.
4.	Janushirasana	05 sec. each side	05 sec.	3 min.
5.	Bhujangasana	05 sec. 3 Turns	05 sec.	30 sec. 6 Turns
6.	Shavasana	30 sec.	10 min.	2 hours

K. For Older People (57 yrs and above.) (VI)

S.No.	Yogasana/ Bandha	Minimum Duration	Fortnightly Increase	Maximum Fortnightly
1.	Paschimottanasana	05 sec.	5 sec.	2 min.
2.	Pawanmuktasana (Lying)	10 sec.	5 sec.	2 min.
3.	Shavasana	1 hour, Twice a day	—	—

I. For Advanced Old Age (VII)

S.No.	Yogasana/ Bandha	Minimum Duration	Fortnightly Increase	Maximum Fortnightly
1.	Pawanmuktasana (Lying)	10 sec.	5 sec.	2 min.
2.	Shavasana	1 hour, Twice a day	—	—

L. One Hour Programme (VIII)

1. Om Dhwani 3 times
2. Gayatri Mantra 1 time with meaning
3. Warm up exercise to open the joints
4. Tadasana
5. Trikonasana
6. Surya Namaskara
7. Shavasana
8. Navasana
9. Kamar Chakrasana
10. Paschimottanasana
11. Konasana
12. Ardha Matsyendrasana/ Vakrasana
13. Vajrasana + Agnisaar Kriya
14. Ustrasana
15. Shashankasana
16. Bhujangasana
17. Shalabhasana
18. Dhanurasana
19. Padottanasana
20. Makrasana
21. Sarvangasana
22. Matsyasana
23. Shavasana
24. Simhasana
25. Hasya Yoga
26. Eye Exercise
27. Pranayama
28. Meditation
29. Prayer for peace.

Note:

- Select the Asanas and perform within 30 minutes.
- Take 5 min. for sinhasana hasya yoga and eye exercise.
- Pranayama 13 min.
- Meditation 10 min.
- Prayer 2 min.

Curative Yogasanas

S.No.	Disease	Yogasanas and Pranayama
1.	Appetite loss	Dhanurasana, mayurasana, sarpasana, mandukasana, yogamudra, pawanmuktasana, chakrasana and agnisarkriya followed by anulom-vilom pranayama.
2.	Asthma	Suryanamaskarasana, sarvangasana, shashankasana, matsyasana, ustrasana, parvatasana bhujangasana, shalbhasana, dhanurasana, gomukhasana, shavasana etc., bhastrika, kapalbhati, suryabhedi pranayama, Neti, jalneti, dhauti.
3.	Arthritis	Tadasana, trikona, suksham exercises of hands and legs, skandhachalan, paschimottanasana. bhujang, shalabha matsyasana, chakrasana, setubandhasana, shavasana, naadishodhan, bhastrika, suryabhedi pranayama.
4.	Anaemia	Yogmudra, paschimottanasana, ardhmatsyendrasana, bhujangasana, sarvangasana, naukasana, pawanmuktasana, dhanurasana. Agnisarkriya, uddiyan bandha, deep breathing and kunjal kriya.
5.	Acidity	Paschimottanasana, yogmudra, bhyjanagasana, surpasana, pawanmuktasana, vajrasana, sarvangasana. Plavini, anulomaviloma uddiyanbandha, kunjal kriya for one week.
6.	Allergy	Vajrasana, ustrasana, ardhamatsyendrasana, gomukhasana, bhujangasana, sarpasana, sarvangasana, matsyasana, singhasana plavini, bhastrika

		nadishodhan and sheetali pranayama; kunjal.
7.	Appendicitis	Paschimottan, shashankasana, sarvang-asana, matsyasana, uddiyan bandha, agnisarkriya, kunjal kriya and enema twice a day.
8.	Backache	Bhujangasana shalbhasana, marjari, ustrasana, makrasana (spine) dhanur-asana, tadasana, pawanmuktasana, ardhmatsyendrasana, vajrasana; Kapal-bhati, agnisarkriya, deep breathing.
9.	Bronchitis	Shashankasana, bhujangasana, ustr-asana, pawanmuktasana, padhastasana, dhanurasana, halasana; Kapalbhati, bhastrika anulom-vilom, kunjal. Neti (both) steam.
10.	Blood Pressure (High)	Tadasana, padhastasana, trikonasana, makarasana (on belly), shithilasana, siddhasana for meditation, pawan-muktasana, badhapadmasana, mandukasana, paschimottanasana, gomukhasana shavasana, Anulom-vilom chand-rabhedi, sheetali pranayama, meditation.
11.	Blood Pressure (Low)	Suryanamaskara, dhanurasana, chakr-asana, (Low) janushirasana, ardh-matsyendrasana, ustrasan, yogmudra, mahamudra. Kapalbhati, bhastrika, anulom-vilom, bhramari, kunjal kriya.
12.	Constipation	Kunjal-shankhprakshalan, Dhanur-asana, sarvangasana, bhujangasana, shalabh, vajrasana, ardhamatsyendr-asana matsyasana, pawanmuktasana,

		janushirasana, gomukhasana; kapalbhati bhastrika, anulom-vilom
13.	Cervical Spondylitis	Bhujangasana, shalabhasana, makarasana (on spine), konasana, dhanurasana, suptvajrasana, tadasana ardha pawanmuktasana, setubandhasana, vakrasana, parvatasana, deep breathing, kapalbhati, anulom-vilom.
14.	Colitis	Tadagimudra, sarvangasana, pawanmuktasana, bhujangasana, shalabhasana, vakrasana, padmasana, shavasana; deep breathing, sheetali, bhramri, yoganidra.
15.	Common cold and cough	Shalabhasana, paschimottanasana, matsyasana, dhanurasana, ustrasana, conasana, suptvajrasana; nadhishodhan, bhastrika; kunjal.
16.	Consumption	Suryanamaskara, shavasana; bhastrika, bhramari pranayama, yoganidra.
17.	Diabetes	Suryanamaskara, dhanurasana, paschimottanasana, mandukasana, ardhmatsyendrasana, yogamudra, mahamudra; kapalbhati, bhastrika, anulom-vilom; kunjal, laghu shankh prakshalana.
18.	Disorders of digestive system	Vajrasana, sarvangasana, paschimott anasana padhastasana, trikonasana, dhanurasana, pawanmuktasana; deep breathing, agnisar kriya; kunjal.
19.	Dysentery	Baddha padmasana, kukkutasana.
20.	Diarrhoea	Pawanmuktasana, vajrasana, shashankasana, shavasana; agnisarkriya, sheetali and ujjai pranayama.

21.	Dyspepsia	Pawanmuktasana, padottanasana, bhujangasana, shalbhasana, halasana, yogamudra, sarvangasana, matsyasana and shavasana; Agnisarkriya, uddiyan-bandha, nauli, anulom-vilom prana-yama.
22.	Drowsiness	Bhujangasana, uttanpadasana, kukkut-asana, bakasana; nadishodhan, bhra-mari pranayama.
23.	Dermatic disease (skin disease)	Yogamudra, paschimottanasana, bhuj-angasana, matsyasana, utkatasana, mandukasana, suptavajrasana; Sheetali, nadishodhan pranayama; kunjal.
24.	Enlargement of liver and spleen	Sarvangasana, halasana, mayurasana, garbhasana, ustrasana, halasana, baddhapadmasana, kamar chakrsana; deep breathing, agnisar kriya, nadi-shodhan pranayama.
25.	Epilepsy	Pawanmuktasana, vipreetkarani mudra, sarvangasana, matyasana, shavasana; Kapalbhati, bhramari, anulom-vilom pranayama–yoganidra, ghrit neti, Neti, meditation.
26.	Feeble mindness	Bhujangasana, tadasana, sarvangasana, suryanamaskara, mahamudra; Nadi-shodhanghritneti, sutra and jal neti–meditation.
27.	Fatigue	Yogamudra, mayurasana, sarvangasana, shithilasana, makarasana (on belly) shavasana. –Deepbreathing, sheetali and sheetkari Pranayama.
28.	Gas troubles	Pawanmuktasana, bhujangtasana, shalbhasana, yogamudra, vakrasana, dhanurasana, shashankasana, paschi-

		mottanasana, vajrasana after meals; Anulom-vilom. Kapalbhati; Kunjal
29.	Hysteria	Shalbhasana, dhanurasana, halasana, sarvangasana; anulom-vilom, nadi-shodhan, kapalbhati, bhramari, ujjai-sutrneti; jalneti.
30.	Headache	Vipreet karani, parvatasana, vakrasana, pawanmuktasana, halasana, sarvangasana, padottasana, yogamudra, dhanurasana, sarpasana and shavasana; Nadishdhan, kapalbhati bhramari; meditation; Kunjal, Neti.
31.	Hernia	Utkatasana, trikonasana, grudasana, sarvangasana, matsyasana, hastpad-ottanasana, suptvajrasana, pawan-muktasana, yogamudra; Deepbreathing, agnisarkriya.
32.	Heart disease	Tadasana, gomukhasana, shithilasana, bhujangasana, padottanasana, makarasana (on spine), shalbhasana, shavasana–Deep breathing, apanvayu-mudra.
33.	Indigestion	Bhujangasana, shalbhasana, yoga-mudra, halasana, sarvangasana, mayurasana, ardha matsyendrasana, shavasana. –Nadishodhan, uddiyanbandha.
34.	Insomnia	Suryanamaskarasana, Shashankasana, janushirasana, dhanurasana, sarvangasana, halasana, matsyasana, parvatasana, paschimottanosana shavasana. –Deep breathing, kapalbhati, chand-rabhedi–meditation, yoganidra.

35.	Jaundice	Bhujangasana, shalabhasana, padottanasana ardha matsyendrasana, –Nadishodhan sheetali–Kunjal.
36.	Kidney disorders	Ardha-matsyendrasana, dhanursana, vajrasana, matsyasana, pawanmuktasana, bhujangasana, shalbhasana, yogamudra, vakrasana, shavasana. –Uddiyanabandha, kapalbhati, bhastrika, anulom–vilom, bhramari–kunjal (saltless)
37.	Leucoderma	Janushirasana, padmasana, siddhasana, gomukhasana, vakrasana, vrikshasana, vipreetkarani, sarvang, matsya, halasana–Agnisar, sheetali, deep breathing uddiyan banddha, nadishodhan–Enema, Kunjal.
38.	Leucorrhoea	Yogamudra, pawanmuktasana, vajrasana, bhujangasana, shalabhasana, makarasana, dhanurasana, padottanasana, vipreetkarani, shalabhasana, suptrajrasana, shavasana. –Nadishodhan, bhastrika by chandra swar, ashivini mudra, uddiyanbandha. –Kunjal kriya. Jalneti.
39.	Lack of memory	Sarvagasana, yogamudra, makarsana, dhanurasana, shavasana. –Nadishodhan pranayama, bhramari, –Gayatrimantra, meditation.
40.	Menstrual disorder	Trikonasana, tadasana, janushirasana, paschimottanasana, suptvajrasana, bhujangasana, shalbhasana, dhanurasana, makrasana (on spine) halasana, sarvangasana, matsyasana, shavasana.

		Note: Don't do the asanas during the periods–Deep breathing, anulom-vilom, pranayama.
41.	Menopause	Janushirasana, ardhamatsyendrasana, ustrasana, yogamudra, suptvajrasana, sarvangsana, dhanurasana, naukasana, sarpasana, pawan muktasana, bhujangasana, shalbhasana, halasana, matsyasana and shavasana–Ujjai, anulom-vilom, bhramari and deep breathing pranayama–meditation.
42.	Piles	Sarvangasana, matsyasana, halasana, sheersasana, mahamudra, gomukhasana siddhasana, paschimottanosana–Nadishuodhan pranayama, ashvini mudra–Enema–Kunjal
43.	Prostate disorder	–Suryanamaskara, pawanmuktasana, sarvangasana, matsyasana, shalbhasana, halasana, paschimottanasana, yogamudra–moolbandha, ashvinimudra, kapalbhati–kunjal
44.	Sciatica	Padmasana, paschimottanasana, gomukhasana, vajrasana, padottanasana, janushirasana, padhastasana, sarvangasana, shavasana–Sheetali pranyama–Kunjal
45.	Tension/stress	Sarvangasana matsyasana, dhanurasana, janushirasana, shashankasana, shavasana–Bhramari pranayama – shanmukhi mudra, Gayatri mantra – meditation, yoganidra.
46.	Thyriod Disorders	Konasana, sarvangasana, matsyasana halasana, greeva chalanamudra,–Ujjai, bhramari pranayama, om sound.

47.	Obesity	Naukasana, dhanurasana, sarpasana, sarvangasana, matsyasana, paschimottanasana kurmasana, chakrasana, ustrasana, suptvajrasana,–Bhastrika –Kapalbhati,–Kunjal, Shankh prakshalana
48.	During pregnancy	Shithilasana, sukhasana, padmasana, tadasana, utkatasana, setubandhasana, ardhahalasana, ustrasana shashankasana, vakrasana –Deep breathing anulom vilom pranayama–meditation

● ● ●

8

Exercises for Flexibility

These exercises are related to anti-rheumatic group and Pawanmuktasana series. They are very useful and light, they can easily be performed. They are called Sukshm vyayama also.

Benefits of Exercises

1. Loosening up the joints of the body.
2. To promote the impeded flow of pran through the nadis primarily by releasing the blockage in the joints.
3. These are excellent for those with rheumatism, arthritis, high blood pressure, heart problems or other ailments where vigorous physical exercise is not advised.
4. These work on the pranic and mental bodies.
5. These are energizational exercises.
6. These are for warming up the body.

Mind these Points

- Never tense with a quick or jerky motion.
- Never exert tension to the point of strain.
- Count the rounds. It induces peace, balance and concentration with the result of harmony in the body.
- Perform these exercises with inhaling position.

- After every activity/movement/definite rounds take rest and normalise the breathing.
- Visualise the cosmic energy entering the body through the medulla oblongata.
- Do these exercises before starting your yogabhyasa-—(Practice of yogasanas) for 10-15 days continuously.
- Mostly these exercises should be performed in the base position and sukhasana.

Types of Exercise

1. **Sitting Position (Base Position/Dandasana):**

Sit with the legs outstretched. Place the palms on the asana just behind the buttocks. The back, neck and head should be erect slightly leaning back taking the support of the arms. Close the eyes and relax the body.

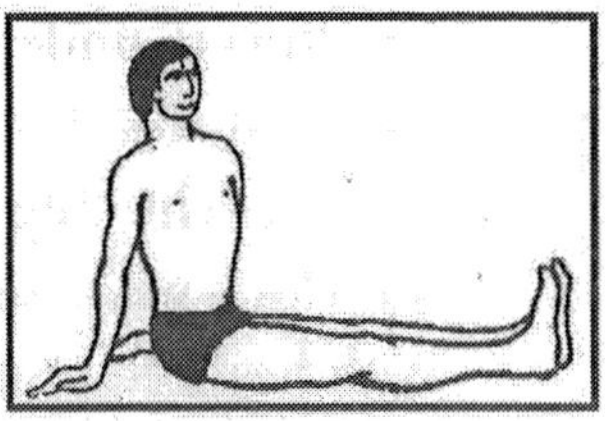

Fig. 52

2. **Toe Bending:**

(a) Inhale and close the fingers for 6 seconds and open for five times or more. Breathing out.

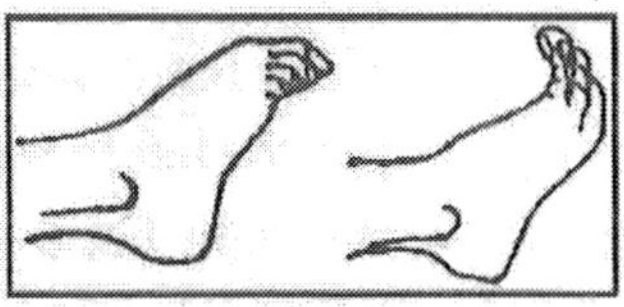

Fig. 53

(b) Inhale and move the toes of both feet slowly backward and forward. Repeat 5 times or more. Breathing out, Relax.

3. **Ankles Rotation:**

Rotate one ankle clock-wise and anticlockwise 5 times or more. Rotate the second ankle. Rotate both the ankles together inhaling position. Breathing out according to the need. Relax.

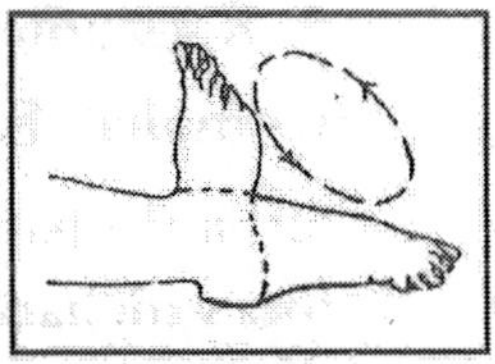

Fig. 54

4. **Ankle Crank:**

Bend the right knee and bring the foot on the joint of left thigh. Hold the upper portion of right ankle with the left hand. Rotate right ankle with the help of left hand. Repeat 5 times or more both sides. Repeat with the left foot placing on the right thigh.

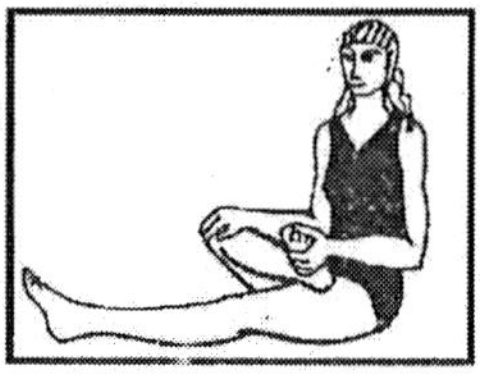

Fig. 55

5. **Knees Rotation:**

Fold the right leg. Interlock the fingers under the thigh lift the foot 3 inches above the ground level. Rotate the leg clock-wise and anticlock-wise, making the big circle with heels. Repeat with the other leg also.

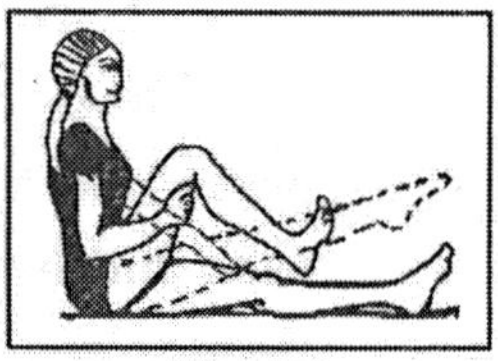

Fig. 56

6. **Hip Joint Rotation (Ardha-Titli Asana):**

1. Sit in basic position. Fold left leg and put the left foot on the right thigh. Put the right hand on right knee and the left hand on the left heel. Twist the leg right and left 5 times and relax. Perform with other leg also.

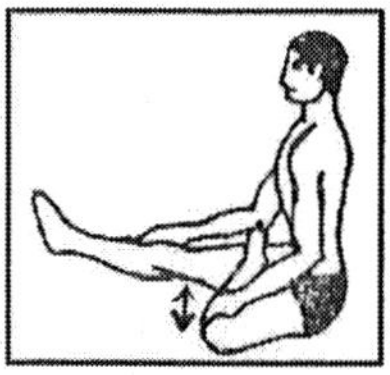

Fig. 57

2. Touch the knee to the ground again and again 5 times and relax. Perform with the other leg.
3. Rotate the knee one by one.

7. **Complete Butterfly Asana (Titli) :**

Sit in the basic Asana. Bring the soles together. Catch the toes with hands. Sit for some time. There will be pain for a short period.

Note:

- Place the hands on the knees. Using the palms, gently push the knees downward towards the floor, and taking up again. Repeat 10 times and relax.

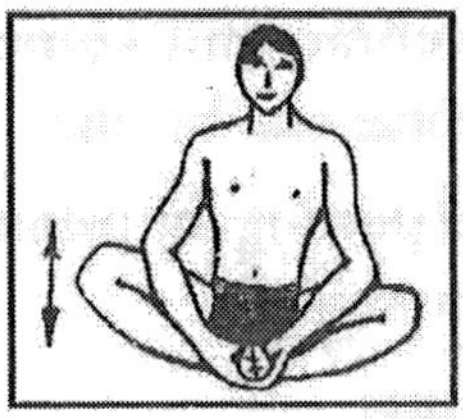

Fig. 58

8. **Crow Walking:**

Squat on the floor, place palms on the knees. Maintaining the squatting position walk on the toes/soles of the feet. Keep the Spine Straight. Walk 1-2 minutes.

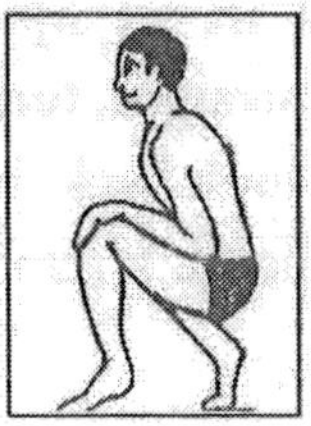

Fig. 59

9. **Rotation of Knees in Standing Position:**

Stand straight. Keep the palms on the knees. Bow the knees downward a bit. Rotate the knees first right side then left side 5-10 times.

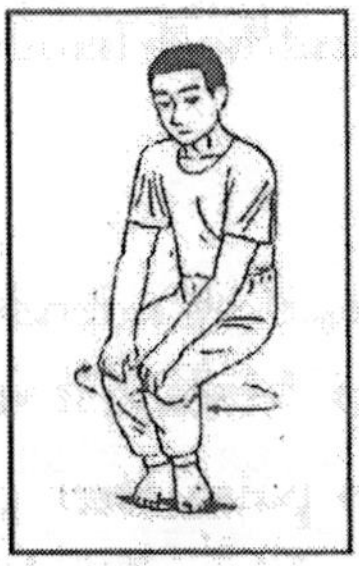

Fig. 60

10. Massage of the Spine:

Stand erect put both the thumbs on the lowerest vertebrae. Press it lightly with inhaling-gradually go on upwards massaging one-by-one vertebrae and come down pressing the vertebrae one-by-one.

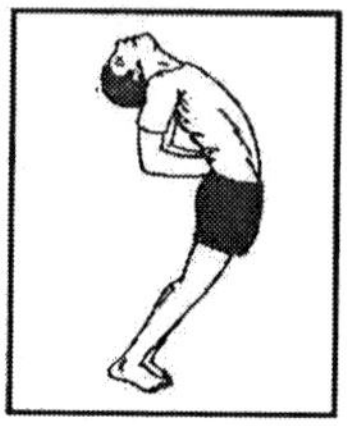
Fig. 61

- Bend backward putting the palms on the waist for one minute.

11. Twisting the Spine:

Stretch both legs wide apart in the front. Bring both the hands and lift upwards in the same level. Then catch the big toe with the right hand and turn the left hand in an upward direction and keep it straight, turn the neck backwards and look back. In the same way repeat the exercise with the left hand. It removes the stiffness of lumber region.

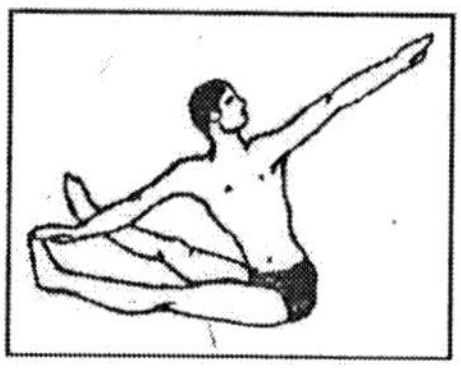
Fig. 62

12. Wrist Bending:

Maintain the starting position, with arms extending forward at shoulder level. Bend the hands back at wrist breathing in. Bend wrist to point fingers down breathing out.

Practice with one hand/both hands. Repeat 10 times.

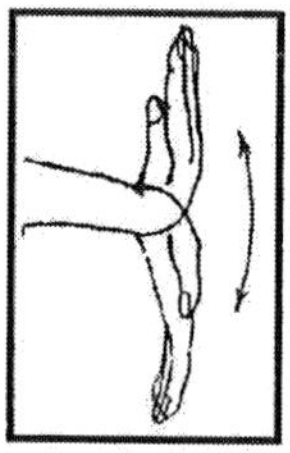
Fig. 63

13. Hand Clenching:

Sitting in starting position, extend arms forward at shoulder level. Bring palm up. Making it vertical. Breathing in.

- Close fingers on palm after culting, creating enough pressure on palm. Make fist. Move like this.

- Open the palm and make fist ten times.
- Rotate the fist clockwise and anticlock-wise 10 times each side.

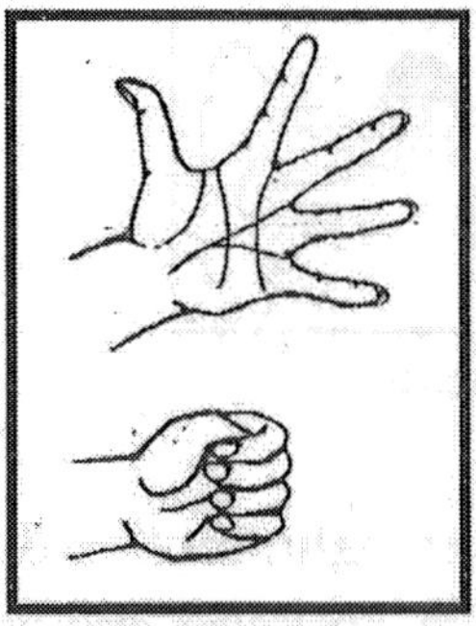

Fig. 64

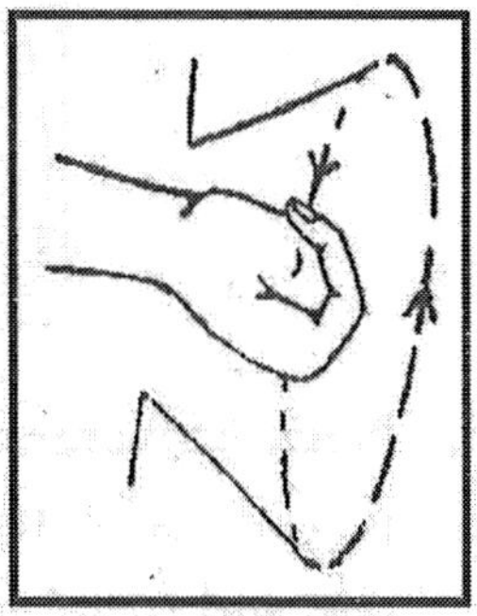

Fig. 65

14. Elbow Bending:

Sit in sukhasana/stand straight. Extend arms forward. Palms turned upwards. Touch the shoulder/with fingers breathing in/Breathing out straighten the arms.

- Repeat some movement extending arms sidewise. Breathing in while bend at elbows. Breathing out while extend the arm. Repeat 10 times.

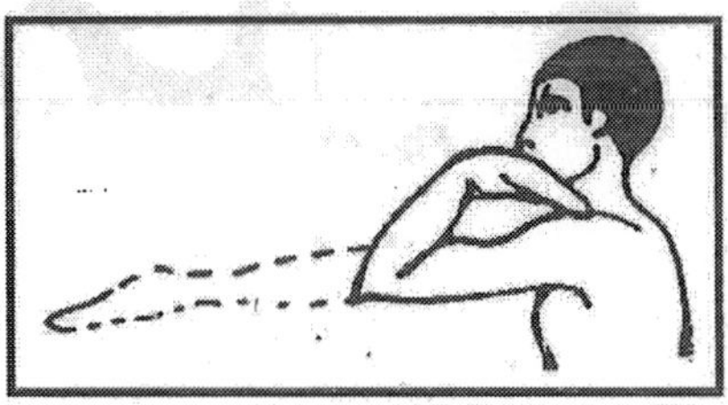

Fig. 66

15. Shoulder Rotation:

Touch the shoulders with fingers. Inhale and move the elbows in a circular pattern rotation shoulders joints (clock-wise) Repeat 10 times Breathing out rotate anticlockwise.

Repeat 10 times making the circular motion as large as possible bringing both the elbows in front of the chest. Rotate all sides also.

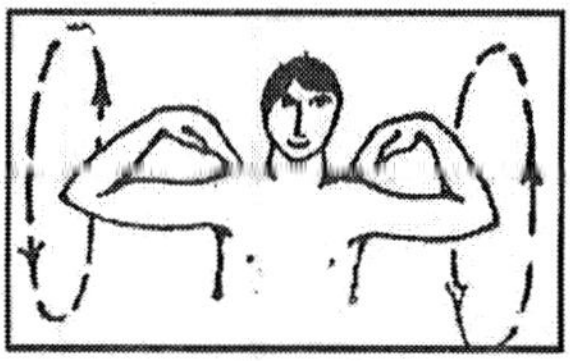

Fig. 67

16. Neck Movements:

Press the neck Forward, straight, backward, right side, left side and rotate in a circle clockwise and anti-clockwise 5 times each.

- Catch the wrists with opposite hands and take them at the back of the head. Inhale and pull the hands right side, left side and back side.

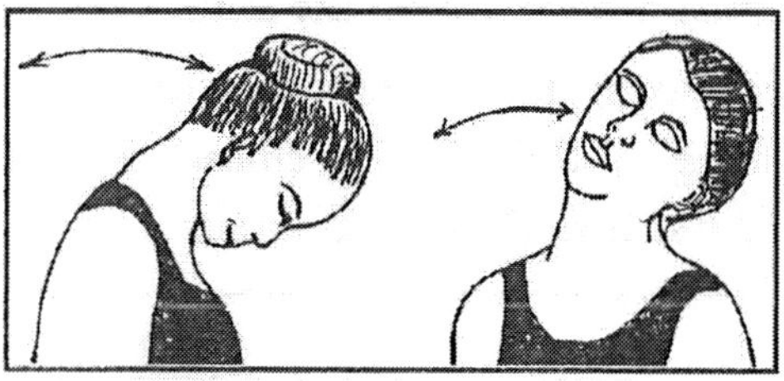

Fig. 68

• • •

9

Yogic Mudras (Yogic Seal)

"Mudra" means a seal. It is because mudra seals the mind with the soul. The exercises of 'mudra' are associated with retention of breath. "Mudras are highly effective to controlling the vital forces (Pranas) and there by controlling the mind for the awakening of the hidden mystic powers, it is the goal of life."

"Mudras awaken the mystic power of kundalini. Success in 'Mudras' enables one to enter into the deeper realms of yoga and to acquire the latent powers of the spirit, 'Mudras' endow one with a magnetic personality, these help in the practice of Brahamcharya (conservation and transmutation of sex-energy), getting powerful will, effulgence in the face, a balanced mind and success in every field of life."

Kinds of Yogic Mudras

In Gherand Samhita 25 mudras are described but 19 are important which are given here.

1. Mahamudra

Method: Sit in the pose of Janushirasana. Perform moolbandha and press the Kanda space between anus and the generative organ by the left heel. Keep the right leg straight. Bend down and hold the big toe of the right foot with both hands. Touch the knee with forehead. Inhale and retain the breath with Jalandhar Bandha (Pressing the chin firmly against the chest).

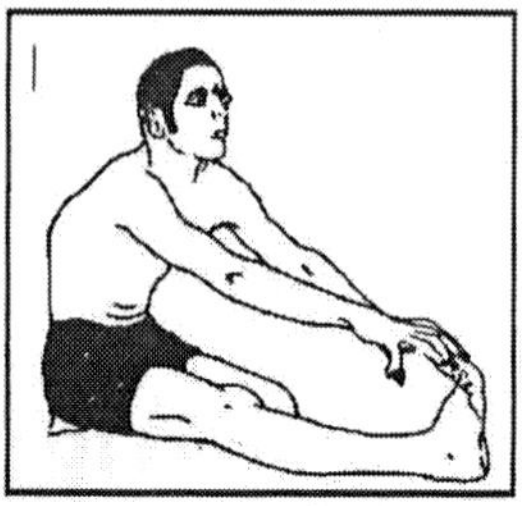

Fig. 69

Exhale while performing **Uddiyan Bandha** (Taking the navel forcibly towards the back). Perform the pranayama as long as possible.

Do the same, keeping the left leg straight and by pressing the **Kanda** with the right heel. Keep the gaze fixed between the eyebrows. Meditate upon the Agya Chakra or on the passage of sushumna naadi (the central mystic channel in the spinal column).

Note: Perform maha bandha and maha bheda after maha mudra.

Benefits:

1. It combines forces of Pran and Apan to pass through the sushumna to arousing the kundalini.
2. It is the key to great sidhis (psychic powers).
3. It purifies the blood.
4. It cures leprosy, piles, gastritis, constipation, consumption and other diseases.
5. It augments digestion and tones up the nervous system.

2. Maha Bandha Mudra (great lock)

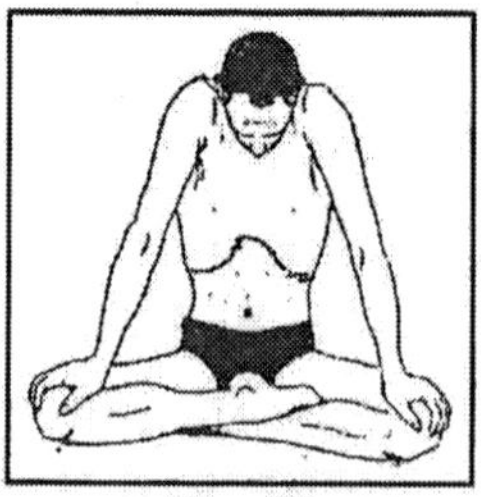

Fig. 70

Method: Sit in half padmasana with the left heel pressing the perineum/vagina and the right foot on top of the left thigh.

Breathe in slowly through the left nostril and perform antrik kunbhak, then observe Uddiyan Bandha, Jalandhar Bandha and

Mool Bandha and Shambhavi Mudra (concentrate between eye brows/Agya Chakra) close the eyes.

Before exhaling release shambhavi mudra than Moolbandha and lastly Jalandhar bandha when the head is upright and the shoulders are relaxed, exhale slowly through the right nostril.

Then breathe in slowly through the right nostril and practise as said above. When exhaling, breathe through the left nostril.

This is one round. Normalise the breath for a minute or two and concentrate on the natural breath. Practise three rounds initially and increase up to five.

Benefits:

1. Stabilises the Pran which controls the mind.
2. It develops the lungs capacity.
3. Mind becomes silent.
4. It develops the concentration power.
5. It cures the respiratory disorders.

Note:

- Practice bandhas separately sometime.
- People suffering from high blood pressure, low blood pressure, hernia, stomach or intestinal ulcer, or those recovering from any visceral ailments will have to correct this condition before attempting mahabandha mudra.

3. Maha Bheda Mudra

Method: Sit in padmasana. Relax the body. Close the eyes. Place the palms on the ground behind the thighs, inhale slowly and deeply through the nose, rotation on the breath and perform Jalandhar Bandha. Raise the body by placing all the weight on the hands. Straighten the arms and gently beat the buttocks on the ground for 3-7 times, keeping your awareness in mooladhar. Then rest the buttocks on the ground, release Jalandhar Bandha, sit quietly and exhale showly and deeply. This is one round. Normalise the breath then again repeat the process. Sit silently after completing the rounds.

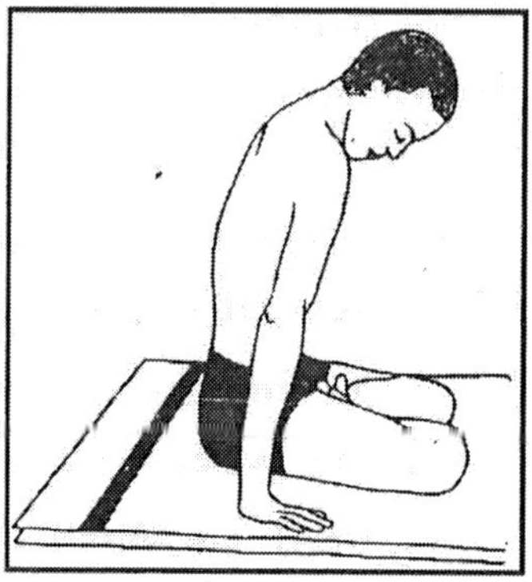

Fig. 71

Practise three rounds in the beginning. After a few months increase up to five but no more.

Benefits:

1. It slows down the aging process.
2. It introverts the mind and awakens psychic faculties.
3. It affects the pineal and pituitary glands and thus the whole endocrinal system.
4. It controls hormonal secretions and regulates them.
5. It bestows abundance of energy and awakens kundalini shakti and leads to the attainment of Samadhi.
6. Mahabhedha is a great purifier of the body and the mind.

Note: Mahamudra, mahabandha and mahavedha (Mahabheda) should be performed during the 3 hours.

4. Yoni Mudra (Shanmukhi Mudra)

Method: Sit in siddhasana. Close both ears with the thumbs, both eyes with the index fingers. Both nostrils with the middle fingers. And the ring fingers above the upper lip and the small fingers under the lower lip. Now inhale and retain the breath. Repeat on and concentrate on Agyachakra (between the eye-brows).

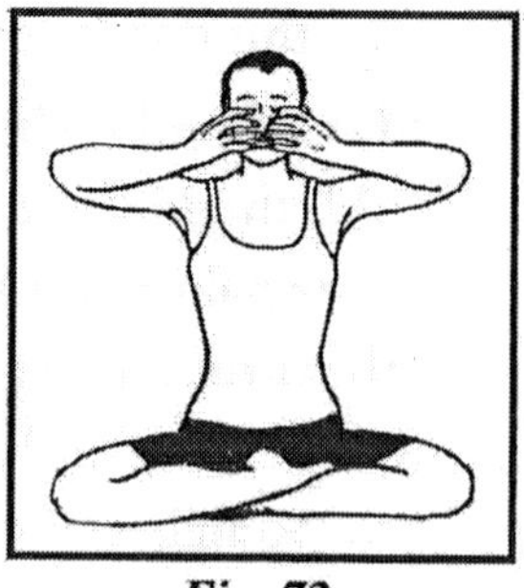

Fig. 72

Perform Mool Bandha and feel that kundalini shakti is ascending the sushumna piercing the six chakras. Exhale and release the fingers.

Benefits:

1. It helps in deep meditation and japa.
2. It awakens the kundalini.
3. It confers great powers of the body and mind.
4. It bestows mental peace and serenity.
5. It stimulates the hearing of the Anahat sounds. These sounds emanate from Bindu.
6. It is good against sufferings from vertigo, eyes-nose-ear and brain infections.

5. Unmani Mudra

Method: Sit in padmasana or siddhasana and steady the mind. Keep the eyes half opened. Fix your mind on the space just a few inches from the eyes. Meditate upon the self that is formless, Nameless and Infinite.

Shut out the senses from all objects of the world, lose your mind in calm meditation. This mudra is an advance sadhana.

Benefits:

1. This mudra bestows peace of mind and reveals the inner glories of the spirit through samadhi.
2. The mind and all the senses become insensitive.
3. The light of knowledge originates and the sadhaka experiences the Truth.

6. Shambhavi Mudra

Method: Sit any meditative pose (padmasana/siddhasana/ sukhasana/swastikasana. Keep your eyes steady looking at Bhrumadhya (Eye brows). Stop the thoughts. Forget the body and surroundings. Let the mind merge in silence.

Benefits:

1. It is highly beneficial for the practice of advanced meditation and samadhi.
2. The Pineal gland is ravitalized.
3. It controls on mind and thoughts.
4. The entrance in spiritual world becomes easy.
5. To cross the difficult path, it is a important method.

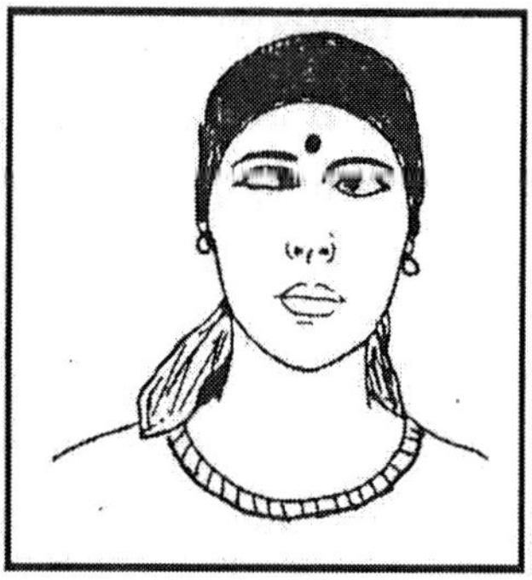

Fig. 73

Note: You can keep the mind in the heart to get peace.

7. Kaki Mudra (Crow Mudra)

Method: Sit in siddhasana or any meditative pose. Make a tube with your lips. Look at the tip of the nose. Inhale through the mouth and exhale through the nose after retaining the breath. Repeat the practice for 3-5 minutes.

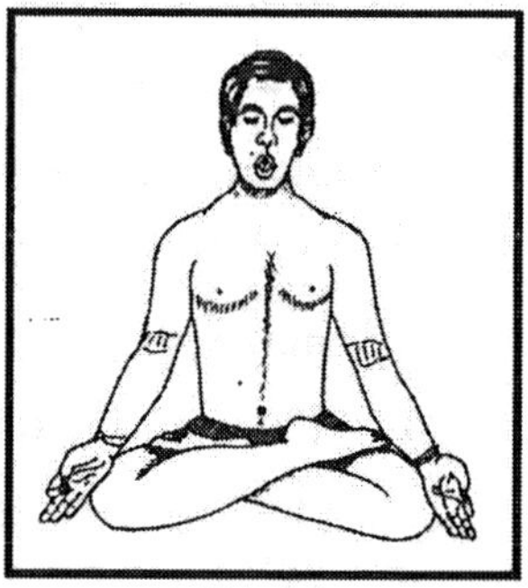

Fig. 74

Benefits:

1. Kaki mudra cools the body and mind.
2. It soothes mental tensions.
3. Alleviating high blood pressure.
4. It purifies the blood.

5. Helps in digestive system.
6. It aids in the development of the mystic vision.

8. Ashwini Mudra

Method: Sit in a comfortable pose, either in sukhasana or in vajrasana. It can be performed in the lying pose, keeping the legs folded in such a way that the heels touch the buttocks.

Contract the anus and release. Do it many times. Repeated contraction and dilation of anus is a wonderful action. It can be practised while sitting or in any other position at any time, any where.

Performing this kriya after doing Bahya kumbhak is more beneficial. Begin with 20 times a minute and increase gradually up to 100 times concentrating on mooladhar chakra.

Benefits:

1. It removes constipation.
2. Sadhak becomes master of Apaan vayu (The vital force that performs excretion).
3. Helps to unfold the mooladhar chakra for the basal plexus.
4. It is beneficial in celibacy and awakening of the pran.
5. It cures the gas, piles and urinary problems and makes the rectum area healthy.
6. Genitals of male and female become healthy and free of problems. The female uterus remains healthy and strong.
7. The delivery of a pregnant woman is performed easily.
8. It is a preparatory practice of 'moolbandha'.
9. It is helpful in prolapse of the uterus/rectum. In such a case. Ashwini mudra is most effectively performed in

conjunction with an inverted asana for example, sarvangasana.

10. It strengthens the anal muscles.

9. Matangini Mudra

Method: It can be done anywhere but river is suitable. Stand in a river. Draw water through nostrils and throw it out through the mouth forming the mouth like a tube and let the water gush forth forcibly. It is similar to Neti Kriya.

Benefits:

1. Matangini mudra tones the optical nerves and the brain.
2. It removes the headache.
3. It prevents from cold.
4. It adds lustre to the face.
5. It paves the way for the attainment of peace of mind.

10. Shakti Chalini Mudra

There are different views about this mudra. According Hathayogapradipica the method is given here.

Method: Sit in siddhasana. Keep the eyes closed. Inhale slowly and deeply through the right nostril and perform antarik kumbhak (retaining breath in side). Perform mool bandha as tightly as possible. Concentrate on the area of contraction. Hold the breath and mool bandha as long as possible. Exhale slowly. Perform Jalandhar and Uddiyan bandha.

Then practise churning nauli, moving the rectum abdomini muscles clock wise in a circular motion from left to right, then directly back to the left and again circling to the right side counting the number of rotations up to ten.

Before inhaling, come back to uddiyan bandha, slowly release uddiyan bandha and jalandhar bandha. Only after the head is raised should inhalation proceed very slowly. This is one round. Do 5 rounds.

Benefits:

1. The problems of laziness, carelessness and stupidity are cured.
2. It awakens the pran very soon, all chakras open and the kundalini awakens.
3. This mudra keeps the uterus and reproductive organs healthy.
4. Destroys the all diseases and brings the radiant health and long life.

11. Tadan Mudra

Method: Sit in padmasana. Inhale and perform Jalandhar and mool bandha and beat the buttocks keeping the palms on the ground.

Benefits:

1. Shakti chalini mudra is associated with Tadan mudra which is done before shaktichalini mudra.
2. It is helpful in awakening the kundalini shakti.

12. Akashi Mudra

Method: Sit in any meditative pose. Fold the tongue against the palate, practise ujjai pranayama and shambhavi mudra.

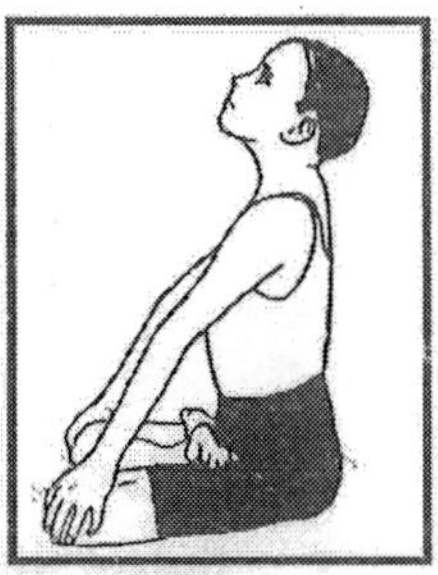

Fig. 75

Benefits:

1. After a long time, it gives the same benefits as khechari.
2. This mudra is very important to prepare for a trance state of mind.

Note:

1. Don't do this mudra if the mind is wandering.
2. In the beginning it irritates the throat.

13. Bhujangi Mudra

Method: Sit in the padmasana/vajrasana. Swallow air in through the mouth and belch it out again. One can keep the air in the intestines for hours. This kriya can be done with smoke also.

Benefits:

1. It cures wind in the intestines and abdominal disorders.
2. It rejuvenates the intestinal organs.
3. It destroys all the chronic diseases.

14. Tadagi Mudra

Method: Sit in paschimottanasana, with feet some what apart, holding the big toes. Inhale while expanding the abdominal muscles. Retain breath and hold this position for five seconds then relax and exhale.

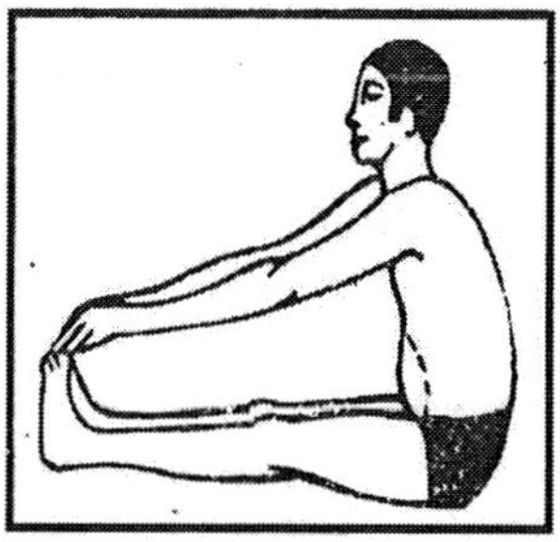

Fig. 76

Benefits:

1. Tadagi mudra relieves any tension stored in the diaphragm and pelvic floor.
2. Tones the abdominal organs.

3. Stimulates blood circulation to these area.
4. It improves the digestion and helps to alleviate diseases of this region.
5. This stimulates manipur chakra the centre of energy.

15. Pashinee Mudra

Method: Practise in Halasana. Bend knees near to shoulders, and entangle them by both arms. Meditate in manipur chakra. Hands should be tight together, as this is the only difference from karn peedasana in which position the arms are free.

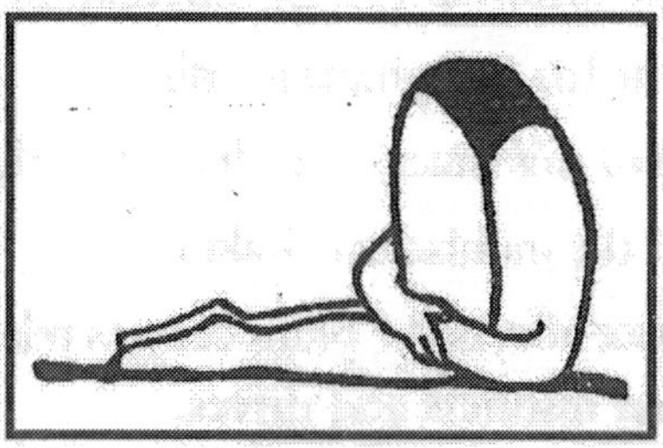

Fig. 77

Relax the whole body in this position and close the eyes. Breathe slowly and deeply. Come back in halasana slowly. Lower the legs and relax in shavasana.

Benefits:

1. Pashinee mudra brings balance and tranquility to the nervous system.
2. It increases pratyahar, sense withdrawal.
3. It stretches the spine and the back muscles and stimulates all the spinal nerves in and around the spine.
4. It massages all the abdominal organs.

16. Manduki Mudra

Method: Sit in vajrasana. Increase the distance between the knees as far as possible. Practice 'Agochari Mudra' gazing at the tip of the nose, holding breath. If the eyes becomes tired relax them. Continue the practice for 5 minutes.

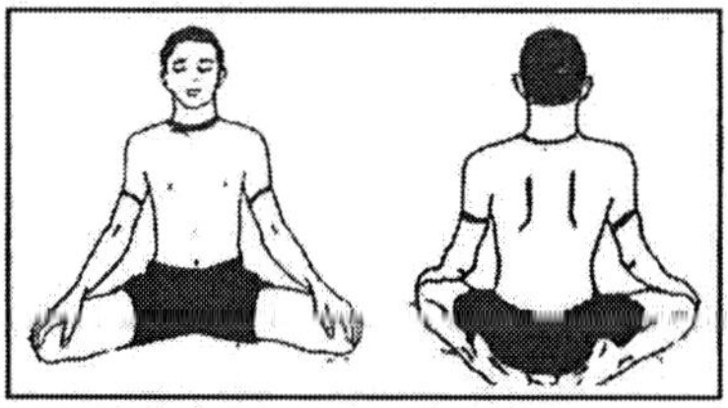

Fig. 78

Benefits:

1. It calms the disturbances and fluctuation of the mind.
2. Balances the Ida and pingla naadis.
3. Perfection of this practice leads to directly to meditation.
4. It awakens the mooladhar chakra.
5. This practice affects the brain centres related to man's most deep rooted instincts and drives.

Note:

- The pose is like a frog sitting in a rest position.
- It is a advanced variation of Nasikagra drishti.
- It should be performed in mild light so that the tip of the nose can be seen.

17. Bhoochari Mudra

Method: Sit in padmasana or any comfortable meditative asana with the head and spine straight and the left hand in chin/ gyan mudra close the eyes and relax the whole body. Open the eyes and raise the right hand flat in front of the nose horizontally. Palm down with all the fingers

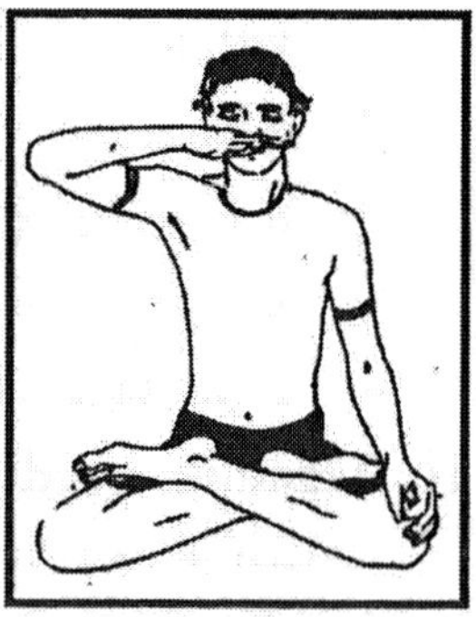

Fig. 79

together. The side of the thumb should be in contact with the top of the upper lip.

Focus the eyes on the tip of the little finger and gaze at it intently for a minute or so without blinking or flickering the eyes. After some time remove the hand but continue to gaze into nothingness at the place. Where the little finger was infront of the face. Try not to blink and think anything. Continue the practice for 5-10 minutes.

Benefits:

1. Bhoochari mudra develops the power of concentration and memory.
2. It tranquillises and introverts the mind.
3. It reduces the anger tendency.
4. All benefits of shambhavi mudra and trataka are achieved.

18. Khechari Mudra

This is a very important mudra. It should be practised under any expert/guru. The name is given: because it produces a state of mind in which the astral body is detached from the physical body. Then, the consciousness dwells in the 'Akash', the space between astral and physical body.

Method: Sit in any meditative asana like padmasana or siddhasana. Spine and head should be straight. Hands in chin/gyan mudra. Relax the body closing the eyes. Fold the tongue upward and backward so that the lower surface lies in contact with the upper palate. Stretch the tip of the tongue backward as far as is comfortable. Perform ujjai Pranayama. Breathe slowly and deeply. Hold for as long as possible. There may be some irritation in the beginning, in the throat. When the tongue becomes tired relax it and repeat the practice again. Practise for 5-10 minutes.

10

Yogic Breathing (Pranayama)

Breathing is the very essence of life. Yet it is hard to believe that so few of us correctly perform something that is as natural as breathing. Most of us breathe shallowly, using only the upper part of our lungs, neglecting, and therefore weakening, the abdominal or lower part of our lungs. The great yoga masters claimed centuries ago. 'He who controls breath, controls life itself.' Today many leading physicians agree that correct breathing, is of vital importance to our health. There is quite a variety of yoga breathing that can help to achieve correct breathing.

What is Pranayama?

"Tasmin Sati Shwasa Prashwasayor Gati vichchedah pranayamah" Yoga Sutra 2/46.

"After the steadiness of Asana or posture, the control of inhalation and exhalation of breath is called pranayama." Pranayama as a process in which respiration is interrupted and pran, that is, the vital force is controlled and regulated. The purpose of pranayama is to inspire, motivate, regulate and balance the vital force (Pran) pervading in the body.

Pranayama is the fourth limb of Astang yoga. It is very important part of yoga. It is the soul of yoga. Pranayama is essential for purifying the mind and nervous system. It is a process of correct breathing to get more energy, peace and long life. It is an exact science. The chief aim of pranayama is to unite Pran with the Apana and take the united pranapana slowly towards the head (Sahasrar chakra) and awakening kundalini.

What is Pran?

Pran is much more than mere breath. Pran is actually the power behind and within breath. The power of the atom is Pran. Thought is pran. It is "the vital force in every being." It is cosmic energy. It pervades the whole universe. It is everywhere and through pranayama we can tap this illimitable well of universal energy.

"In this body of ours the breath motion is the 'Silken thread', by laying hold of and learning to control it we grasp the pack thread of the nerve currents, and from these the stout twine of our thoughts, and lastly the rope of pran, controlling which we react freedom."

–Swami Vivekananda

Pran is the subtlest form of energy that underlies all physical energies such as electricity, magnetism, light, heat etc., and also sustains all mental process such as thinking, feeling, willing and reasoning. Pran is the universal store house of energy. Pran is the manifestation of the supreme spirit, as the sustainer of life and forces in this world.

It is due pran that the ocean surges, the sun shines in the heavens, the stars move along their definite orbit round the sun. It is due to Pran that rivers flow towards the sea and mountains hold their heads high in the air. Without pran there would be no life on earth, there would be no existence of any object. Without pran nothing can exist. This is the meaning of pran in a broader sense.

In a restricted sense pran is the vital force that sustains the life of man by performing various vital functions and keeping the body alive. Breathing is an effect of the pran. By controlling the breath and by harmonizing it a yogi gains control over the subtle Pran. This subtle Pran is linked to the mind and senses. Senses and mind follow the movements of Pran. If Pran departs the senses and mind also leave the body of man. Mind is linked to the soul. The pranic body infuses energy into the physical body.

Parts of the Pran

Pranic energy can be divided into five main pranas according to location and functions–apan saman, pran, udan and vyan.

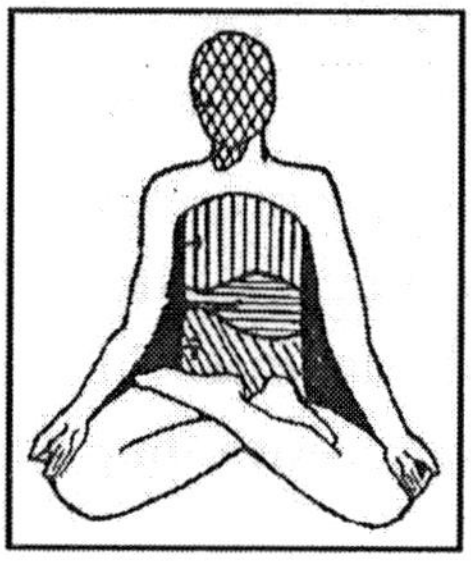

Fig. 80

1. Apan (Below the Navel):

Apan throws out impurities via process of elimination and expulsion. The earth element predominates and thus apan is characterised by heaviness and a downward movement. It results in defecation, urination, ejaculation, menstruation and expulsion of the fetus. Apan aids the flow of digestive juices in the intestines and puts undigested matter towards the anus in the same way a magnet attracts iron. Apan also aids locomotion from the hips to the toe. The colour of apan is yellow or smoky. In terms of digestion, these two aspects of energy function in co-ordination with the other pranas.

2. Saman (From the Navel to the Diaphragm):

Saman activates and controls the digestive system–stomach, liver, pancreas and small intestines. It promotes the secretion of juices and the assimilation of nutrients. Saman is the force/energy which prepares the rasa (essence) or juice of food and distributes it to the respective places in the body, for example, to the nervous system, brain, heart, etc.

3. Pran (Diaphragm to Throat):

Pran creates hunger and thirst, moves food from mouth to stomach and maintains body heat. The fire element is dominant giving it a colour of gold and an upward movement. It is associated with the respiratory system and speech, and the gullet together with the muscles and nerves that activate them. It is the force by which the breath is drawn inside.

4. Udan (Throat and Above):

Udan functions in the process of vomiting and belching, as it is the upward force that keeps the body upright. Associated with air it is blue-green in colour. It controls eyes, nose and ears. Thoughts and consciousness of the outside world would be impossible without it.

5. Vyan (Whole Body):

Vyan keeps the sensory nerves active, thus helping us to perceive and taste. It aids circulation of nutrients in the blood, lymph, etc and performs all functions of the body. Associated with ether it is sky-blue in colour. Vyan pervades in the whole body, regulating and controlling all movements and co-ordinating the other pranas. It acts as the reserve force for the other pranas.

There are five Sub-pranas.

1. **Devadatta (Nostrils):** Yawning and sneezing.
2. **Krikal (Throat):** Yawning, hunger and thirst.
3. **Kurma (Eyelids):** Wrinkling, eyelids movements.
4. **Naga (Mouth):** Belching and hiccup.
5. **Dhananjaya (whole body):** Swelling, movement, nourishment.

Life-style has a profound impact on the pranayama kosha and its pranas. Physical activities such as exercise, work, sleep, intake of food and sexual relations all affect the distribution and flow of the pran in the body. Emotions, thoughts and imagination effect the pranic body even more. Lack of pran caused diseases. Pranayama balances pranas.

Cycles of Pran

Mostly people don't know about pranic clock of their body. If they do according to that they can be healthy. The pranas are working best according to this table.

Largest Pran	Lowest Pran
1. Lungs 3-5 a.m.	7. Bladder 3-5 p.m.
2. Large intestine 5-7 a.m.	8. Kidneys 5-7 p.m.
3. Stomach 7-9 a.m.	9. Heating components 7-9 p.m.
4. Spleen 9-11 a.m.	10. Metabolic process 9-11 p.m.
5. Heart 11- am - 1 p.m.	11. Gall Bladder 11 -p.m. -1 a.m.
6. Small intestine 1-3 p.m.	12. Liver 1-3 a.m.

This list indicates the times when prana is present in the largest quantity in the organs. If the morning meal is taken between 7-11 a.m. and evening meal should be taken before sunset.

Nadis

There are 72000 nadis in our body but three are very important. Ida (left nostril, cold) pingla (right nostril, hot). Susumna when the pran flows from the both nostrils. There are five elements mixed in each pran we must purify the nadis through pranayama and shatkarmas. We take 21600 'Swasa' per day. We can lessen them by pranayama controlling the pran.

Pranic Table

Name	Seat	Function	Colour	Chakra	Result of Control
Main Pran	Heart	Respiration Converting food into vital fluid	Gold	Anahat	Control of mind.
Apan	Below navel	Section of the faecal matter, urine Exhalation of breath.	Yellow/smoky	Mooladhar	Mastery over decay and death.
Saman	Navel to diaphragm	Assimilation and distribution of food	Glossy white	Manipur	Radiant health and abundance of energy.
Udan	Throat and above	Give lightness to the body. It separates the astral body from the physical body	Blue-green	Vishuddhi	Mastery over elements
Vyan	Whole body	Blood circulation	Skyblue	Swadhisthan	Peace of mind poetic ability abundance of energy.

Importance of Pranayama

1. The practice of pranayama is a boon for all. When one has attained mastery over pran, one automatically acquires control over mind, sex, energy, and subtle desires.
2. By constant practice of pranayama one can acquire an abundance of power, miracles can be performed.
3. Control of the vital force leads to the control of the subconscious mind. One can attain immense powers of the spirit.
4. Pranayama provides calmness of mind strength and cheerfulness.
5. Pranayama keeps the body fit and healthy. It reduces excessive fat.
6. One can live a long life through pranayama.
7. It improves the power of memory and eliminates mental disorders.
8. Pranayama tones up the stomach, the liver, the bladder, the small and the large intestines and the digestive system.
9. Pranayama purifies tubular channels and removes sluggishness from the body.
10. Pranayama kindles gastric fire, the body becomes light, clear and the inner voice begins to be heard.
11. It develops the concentration power.
12. Nervous system becomes strong.
13. Constant practice of pranayama rouses spiritual powers. Kundalini shakti awakens.
14. Lungs become strong.
15. Energy is maintained in the body according to the need of the body.
16. We intake more oxygen and carbondioxide goes out.

17. The all round development occurs of peneal and pituitary glands.
18. Tension gets removed.
19. It is helpful in meditation.
20. It increases tolerance, will power and self-confidence.
21. It brings freshness and removes laziness.
22. It is helpful in sound sleep.
23. Pranayama develops the seminal energy.
24. Pranayama nullifies the effect of heat or cold.

Mechanism of Breathing

Our body is a wonderful machine having many different systems. Working harmoniously and in an integrated manner. Our life activity depends more on the respiratory system. We should know about this system.

Ordinary/Normal Breathing

Our normal breathing takes place when the diaphragm contracts, the ribs are elevated and the thorax expands the lungs also expand. Consequently the volume of the thorax increases. When the volume increases, the pressure in the thorax decreases as compared to the atmospheric pressure and the air is drawn in the lungs. This is **inhalation.**

When the pressure in the thorax and atmospheric pressure equalises and thorax does not expand any more, there is pause. This can't go on for a long time. The diaphragm relaxes the ribs sink down and the thoracic cavity decreases. This reduces the volume of the thorax. When the volume is reduced, the pressure in the thorax increases as a result of which the internal air is driven out. That is what we call **exhalation.**

When the ribs can't sink in any further and the thorax can't contract any longer, there is a pause. There are the phases of our normal breathing. In this the diaphragm plays the most important part. The importance of the diaphragm muscle is rarely understood but in many disorders the function of the diaphragm is disturbed.

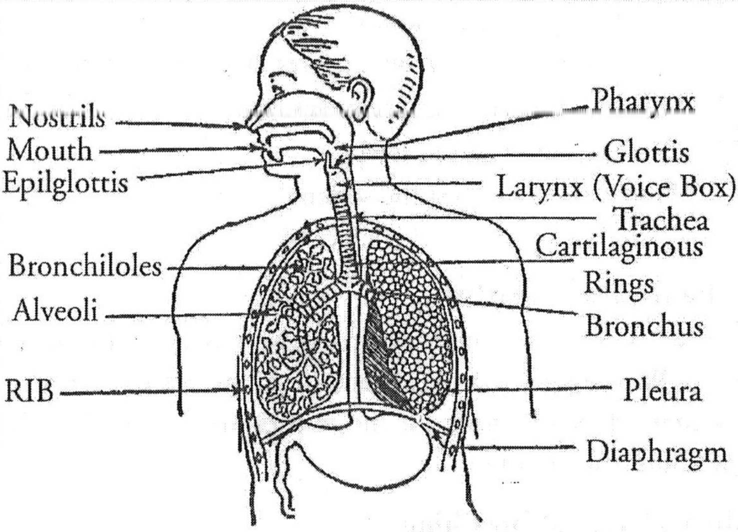

The human respiratory system

Fig. 81

Our respiration is affected by three factors.

1. Biological Factor: The metabolic changes that occur in the body influences respiration. For example, when one runs, one need not adjust the breathing. It is automatically adjusted. Any exertion on the part of the body accelerates breathing automatically. It is like a regulator in an air conditioner or a refrigerator which automatically switches off and on at appropriate time.

2. Emotional Factor: When one is in the grip of emotion depending upon the nature and intensity of emotion, the pattern of respiration changes. In sobbing, the respiration is brief and jerky. When in gay mood or laugh the respiration changes again. When depressed the respiratory pattern differs.

3. Volition Foctor: It means that respiration is influenced at will. Talking, singing where one prolongs breath, are the actions done under volition one can change or modify his breathing within certain limits. This factor is used in pranayama. One is consciously regulating his breathing in pranayama.

Breathing Phases in Pranayama

Breathing in Pranayama is willingly controlled. There are three phases of respiration in pranayama.

1. **Puraka:** Controlled inhalation.
2. **Kumbhaka:** Holding the breath. Inner and Outer.
3. **Rechaka:** Controlled exhalation.

As compared to the normal breathing each phase of respiration is prolonged. In normal breathing rate of inhalation and exhalation is approximately 15 per minute. This means each cycle of inhalation and exhalation takes 4 seconds. In pranayamic breathing the rate of respiration is 2 or 3 which includes about 5 seconds for inhalation, 10-20 seconds for retention and 10 seconds for exhalation.

During inhalation and exhalation of pranayama breathing is done against resistance by narrowing the passage of respiration. By offering resistance to breathing in pranayama, the circulation of blood in the lungs is increased and oxygen in the air is assimilated in the blood.

In pranayama one neither intakes more air nor absorbs more oxygen as compared with normal breathing. If we consider that during every normal inhalation, we take 500 ml of air and if we take normal respiration as 16 per minute then air inspired in normal breathing per minute will be 500 ml × 16 = 8 litres at the rate of 20% oxygen in the atmospheric air the oxygen content in the normal inhaled air per minute will be 1.6 litres. In pranayama breathing where inhalations, retentions and exhalations are practiced 2 per minute approximately and if every deep inhalation draws in 2500 ml air, then the total quantity of air inhaled would be 2500 ml × 2 = 5 litres and oxygen content in it would be 1 litre, this is much less than the contents of our normal breathing. Pranayama efficiently improves the function of the respiratory system. It improves the oxygen intake capacity also.

In pranayama one does not exhale through mouth. Exhalation through mouth. The retention phase gradually gets increased. Beginners practice only controlled inhalations and exhalations. Every phase has to be very smooth and slow.

In kumbhaka three bandhas are used. Kumbhaka works in two ways-inner kumbhaka and the outer kumbhaka. The importance of kumbhaka lies in its psychological and spiritual effects.

Instructions for Pranayama

For effective and proper practice one should strictly follow the following points:

1. Pranayama should be practised in a clean, airy, peaceful place with charming atmosphere.
2. The best time for practice is the early morning. If it is not suitable one can do in the evening.
3. Put the clothes according to the season. Tight clothes should be avoided.
4. A place lashed by strong wind should be avoided.
5. Practice should be done only with an empty stomach. Perform it four hours after the meals and half an hour before meal.
6. Clear the bowels. Take bath. Perform asanas then do the pranayama.
7. Choose the suitable posture like-padmasana, siddhasana, swastikasana, sukhasana, vajrasana. First two are recommended. Spine should be erect and posed steadily.

8. Don't practise pranayama if you feel exhausted. First relax and then do the pranayama.
9. Don't take bath just after the practice of pranayama. Rest for half an hour before taking bath.
10. Practice of pranayama should be increased in winter (September to March). But in summer (April to August) it is advisable to keep up the momentum of the same practice as has been done in winter.
11. Persons whose disposition is dominated by the nature of wind (vaata) should not practice sheetali and sheetkari pranayama, and those dominated by the nature of bile (Pitta) should avoid Suryabhedi and Bhastrika pranayama.
12. Patients suffering from asthma, high blood pressure and hypertension should not practise kumbhaka.
13. Surya Bhedi, Bhastrika should be practised in winter only. Sheetakari and Sheetali should be practised in summer only.
14. One should inhale and exhale slowly and rhythmically during the practice of pranayama. Rhythmic and slow breathing makes the mind steady and calm.
15. A beginner of pranayama should practise inhaling and exhaling only for a few days. The ratio of inhaling (Pueraka) and exhaling (rechaka) should respectively be 1:2. This means that the time spent in exhaling should be double the time spent in inhaling.
16. The time for retention of the breath (Kumbhaka) should be increased gradually, in the first month complete 20 rounds only in inhalation and exhalation. In the next month start retention for four/five seconds only; complete 20 rounds gradually. After this easy going practice increase kumbhaka 8/10 seconds. After 15 days or one month. Kumbhaka should be 12/15 seconds. Like this take next step 16/20

seconds the ratio 1:4:2 is the final keep in mind your capacity.

17. While inhaling, retening and exhaling the breath one must not experience any feeling of suffocation or as a strenuous effort.
18. Maintaining the ratio count om/pranayama mantra 'Om bhuh, Om Bhuvah, Om Swah, Om Maha, Om Janah, Om Tapah, Om Satyam'. This mantra takes 5 seconds. If you are interested in gayatri mantra, you can apply that too.
19. To achieve quick results in pranayama observe celibacy and take sattvic and balanced diet.
20. Take milk and Badam (almond) after practice. Take ghee in meals.
21. In case of sweat instead of wiping it with a towel, massage the body with the hands.
22. Four folded blanket should be spread on the 'Asan' and a white cotton sheet upon it. The body should be warmed up. It is better to clean the white sheet every day.
23. A sound and supple body is a must for the successful practice of pranayama.
24. Never give a break to the practice of pranayama.
25. Give a little rest to the breathing process after every type of pranayama. Discontinue the practice if the respiratory system is not in order or if the breathing process is not smooth.
26. Surya bhedhi pranayama is helpful in alleviating the ailments caused by the nature of wind (vaata). Ujjai pranayama cures those caused by phlegm (Kapha) and Sheetali and Sheetkari help curing those of the bile (pitta). But Bhastrika and Kapalbhati cures diseases caused by all the three humours.

27. Before you sit for practising pranayama, thoroughly clean the nostrils well.
28. You can take a small quantity of fruit juice or a small cup of milk even before the practice. When you finish the practice take a cup of milk or light tiffin after 10 minutes.
29. If there is heat in the brain/head, apply Amla oil or butter on the head before you take bath. Take 'Misri Sharbat' by dissolving sugar candy in water. Do sheetali pranayama also.
30. Perform at least 15 minutes practice daily in the beginning regularly for long time.

Four Methods of Respiration

The yogis classify respiration into four general methods, viz.

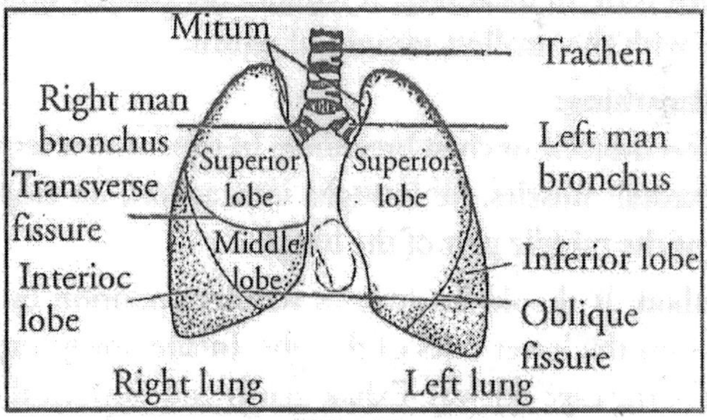

Fig. 82

1. **High Breathing** (Clavicular/coller-bone/upper part Breathing)
2. **Mid Breathing** (Costal/Thoracic/Rib/Chest Breathing)
3. **Low Breathing** (Abdominal/Deep/Diaphragmatic Breathing)
4. **Complete Breathing** (Yogic Breathing)

   There are three parts of lungs. First three methods are according/the parts.

1. High Breathing:

In this form of breathing, the smallest and the upper most part of the chest and lungs is used, and consequently, only a small amount of air enters in the lungs. The best way to open out and ventilate this part is.

Method: Sit in vajrasana. Stretch the arms straight up, then fold them and place the palms on the upper back. Breathing in this position will be shallow and the upper part of the lungs–the apex-will naturally come into action.

Benefits: The apex of the lungs is often the most neglected and it contains most of the locked, residual air. It is often the breeding place for diseases like T.B. Hence, it is necessary to activate this part of the lungs. But high breathing, when done singularly, as a habit, is the worst form of breathing. It requires the greatest expenditure of energy with the smallest amount of return.

2. Mid Breathing:

This is thoracic or chest breathing. In this form of respiration, the Intercostal muscles are brought into action, developing the capacity of the middle part of the lungs.

Method: It should be done in standing position by placing the hands on the lower sides of the ribs. Inhale slowly, expanding the chest or the cage sideway. Exhale gently and contract the ribs in wards. No effort or force should be used by the hands. Immediately after inhaling exhale and let your lungs come back to the normal position. When mastery is gained, while exhaling, slight effort can be made to remove the dead air from the lungs by a slight force as if squeezing the lungs, white wings.

Benefits: It increases the capacity of lungs. It may also be a preventive as in asthma. It re-energises the body and increases mental concentration.

3. Low Breathing (Abdominal Breathing):

This form of respiration is also known as diaphragmatic or deep breathing.

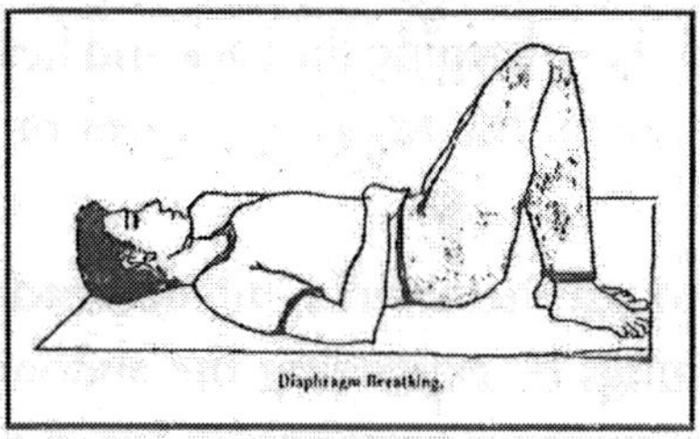

Fig. 83

Method: It is the best done in a lying position to start with. Place one hand lightly on the navel so that the abdominal movements may be felt. Inhale deeply and the hand will rise as the diaphragm flattens, pushing and abdominal contents down and making the stomach expand. The diaphragm, which is the main muscle used in respiration, is strong and large and it separates the lungs from the abdominal organs. The lower pit moves during inhalation, the greater is the expansion of the lungs. Therefore, more air is inhaled into them. Now exhale deeply and notice how the hand moves down on the abdomen. If you try to account this contraction a little, the diaphragm will move higher and more air is expelled out of the lungs. The whole process is as if you are breathing with the stomach expanding it gradually when inhaling and contracting it while exhaling. The chest and shoulders do not move. Of all the three, this is the best type of breathing. If you breathe your stomach you will never fall ill.

4. The Complete Breathing (Yogic Breathing):

After the above training you are now ready to take the deepest breath of your life—the complete Breath, which is the way every one should really breathe. It is a combination of high, mid and low breathing, making it possible to inhale the optimum amount of air into the lungs and also to exhale the maximum amount of waste air.

Method: Sit on the floor in one of the meditative posture or sit in a straight-backed chair, keeping the back and head erect, the hands cupped on the lap or on the respective knees or lay down on the floor.

Breathing through the nostrils, inhale steadily first filling the lower part of the lungs by expanding the abdomen. Then fill the middle part of the lungs by pushing the lower ribs outwards and broadening the chest. Finally, fill the upper part of the lungs by protruding the upper chest. The shoulders may be slightly elevated. In the final movement, the lower part of the abdomen will be slightly down in. This is one inhalation. Though it is visualised as having three stages, there should be one continuous wavelike movements.

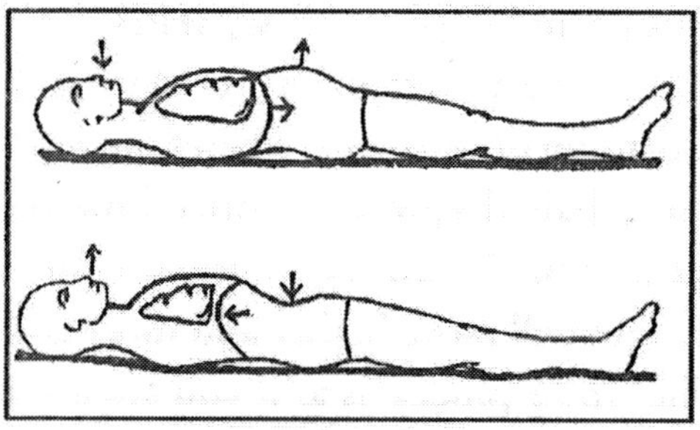

Fig. 84

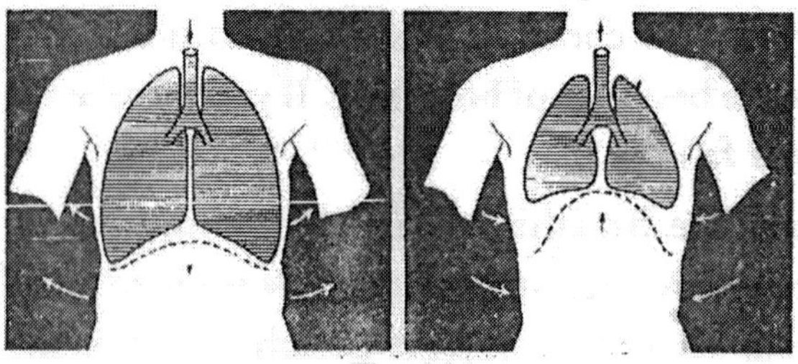

Fig. 85

Exhale slowly in a similar, controlled movement. Holding the chest in a firm position and drawing the abdomen in, gradually lift it upward as the air leaves the lungs. Then relax the chest as the ribs contract and the collar bone is lowered.

Try to follow this procedure for every respiration. You will be amazed to find what a large lung capacity you have and how little it was being used. Do it for a few minutes.

Benefits:

1. It decreases cough, flue, bronchitis, asthma, cardiac troubles, and high blood pressure diseases.
2. Vigorous breathing will spread a glow all over the body.
3. Most cold can be cured by the complete breath and partial fasting for a day.
4. Vitality increases tremendously and one does not tire easily.
5. It increases thinking power as stress, anxiety and melancholia decreases.
6. It is like a complete transformation in the personality.
7. Complete Breathing is of vital importance to every man, woman and child who wishes to be healthy.

Three Types of Pranayama

There are three types of pranayama, viz.

1. **Adham Pranayama:** Consists of 12 matras (seconds)
2. **Madhyam Pranayama:** Consists of 24 matras (seconds)
3. **Uttam Pranayama:** Occupies a time 32 matras (seconds) Matra means measurement of Puraka Time 1 Om is called one matra.
    - Practise for one month the Adham Pranayama.
    - Practise for three months the Madhyam Pranayama.
    - Practise the Uttam Pranayama.

Final ratio should be 16: 64: 32.

Breathing (Pranic) Exercises

These are simple exercises to learn and practice the pranayama.

Exercise No. 1

Sit in sukhasana or any meditative posture. The body should be kept perfectly steady with head, neck and back in a straight line. Close the right nostril with the right thumb and slowly inhale through the left nostril as long as you can with ease and comfort. Then exhale through the same nostril. Do this at least 10 times. This will constitute the first round. To begin with two such rounds must be done daily and increased up to 12 rounds gradually.

Inhale through the right nostril by closing the left nostril with the little and ring finger of the right hand just in the same manner as done before. Then exhale through the same nostril. This must be done at least 2 to 12 times.

Exercise No. 2

Sit in the same posture. Close the right nostril with the right thumb and inhale through the left nostril. Then close the left nostril with the little and ring fingers of the right hand and exhale through the right nostril after removing the thumb. Inhaling again through the right nostril and closing it with the thumb. Exhale through the left nostril. Repeat it at least 10 times.

Exercise No. 3

Sit in the same sitting posture, inhale through both the nostrils as much as you can with ease and comfort and exhale through both the nostrils in the same manner. Do it atleast 10 times and increase the number gradually.

Exercise No. 4

Sit in the same sitting posture, draw the air in through the both nostrils, retain it as long as you can with ease and comfort, then exhale slowly. This process may be repeated 12 times. This will constitute on round and the number of such rounds may he increased gradually.

Exercise No. 5

Sit in meditative pose. Meditate that the single letter, the Supreme light—the Pranava/Om-is the origin or source of these three letters A.U.M., Inhale the air through the left nostril for the space of 16 matras (16 seconds), meditate on the letter 'A (8)' during the time; retain the air for the space of 64 matras (seconds), meditate on the letter 'U (ɫ)' during the time; Exhale through the right nostril for the space of 32 matras (seconds) and meditate on the letter 'M (;)' during the time. Practise this again and again in the above order. Begin with 2 or 3 times and gradually increase the number to 20 or 30 times according to your capacity and strength. To begin with, keep the ratio 1: 4: 2, gradually increase the ratio to 16: 64: 32.

Exercise No. 6

It is 'Pacifying Breath'. Sit in meditative pose, close the eyes and concentrate the mind on breathing.

1. Inhale counting six, Exhale counting six, continue this slow rhythm trying to suspend all thoughts.
2. Inhale counting. 6
   Hold the breath counting 3
   Exhale counting 6
   Retain emptiness, counting 3

Benefits: The slow and rhythmic tempo has great power to relax and pacify the mind and the whole nervous system.

Bandhas (Locks)

1. Mool Bandha:

Contracting the anus, draw upwards the Apan vayu slowly by practice, is called Mool Bandha. It can he usefully practised by sitting in any meditative pose or standing.

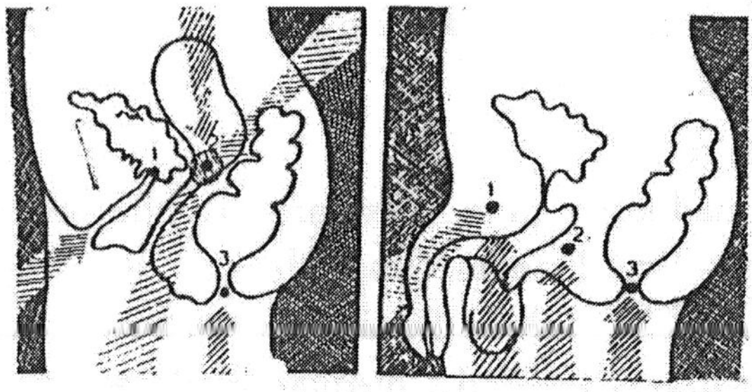

Fig. 86

Benefits:

- Gaining control over the elementary canal.
- Removes the weakness of the excretory system.
- Modifies our animal desires.
- Maintains the celibacy.
- Kindles gastric fire.
- Eliminates constipation and nourish virility.
- It awakens the kundalini.
- It helps in keeping youth for a long time.
- Our nerves breath and feelings are brought under control.

2. Uddiyan Bandha:

This bandha can be practised in either standing position or in a sitting pose of padmasana. Place the hands slightly on the knees, exhale with full force. Contract the abdomen and pull it upwards and backwards to the spine with force of the navel and the diaphragm. It is practised with 'Kumbhaka' after Rechaka. In mahabandha it is locked after mool bandha and unlocked first.

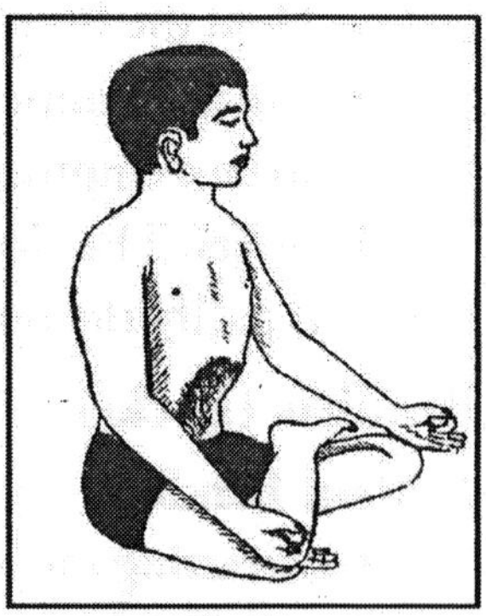

Fig. 87

Benefits:

- It awakens kundalini shakti.
- It preserves the celibacy.
- Makes the body vigorous and healthy.
- It is helpful in Agnisar and Nauli kriya.
- Seminal energy ascends towards the Brahm Randhra.

3. Jalandhar Bandha:

Sit in any meditative posture. Contract the neck and the throat (glottis) and bend the head low. Press the chin firmly against the chest. In mahabandha it is locked in the end and unlocked atfer Uddiyan Bandha.

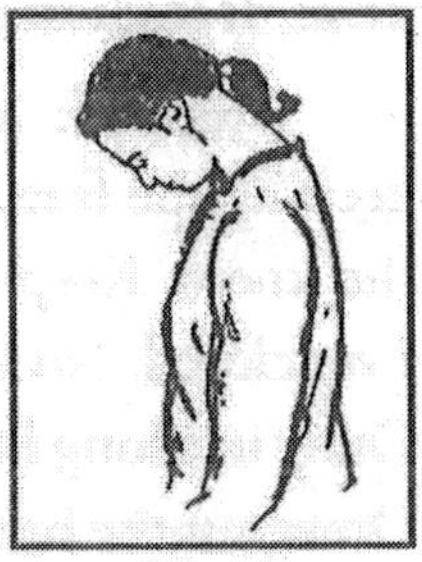

Fig. 88

Benefits:

- Closes the Ida and Pingla nadis.
- Sublimates kundalini shakti.
- Pran begins to flow in its proper channel.
- It is practised along with external or internal kumbhaka.
- It enhances the capacity of retaining the breath for longer period and uniting the pran with Apanvayu.

Mahabandha: All the three Bandhas are performed with external and internal kumbhaka is in Bhastrika and Kapalbhati.

Kinds of Pranayama

1. Deep Breathing:

It is a basic exercise of inhalation and exhalation. Each deep breathing consists of a very full inhalation through the nose and a deep; steady exhalation also, through the nose.

Method: Sit in a meditative posture. First exhale and use a light Uddiyan Bandha and Mool Bandha. Inhale slowly and deeply.

Let the belly come out. Exhale slowly, let the belly come in side. Like this practise 3 to 5 minutes. Concentration will be on breathing. or Navel (nabhi manipur chakra).

2. Agnisar Kriya:

This is very effective pranayama for digestive system. It reduces obesity, cures constipation, helps in performing the Nauli kriya. It increases appetite.

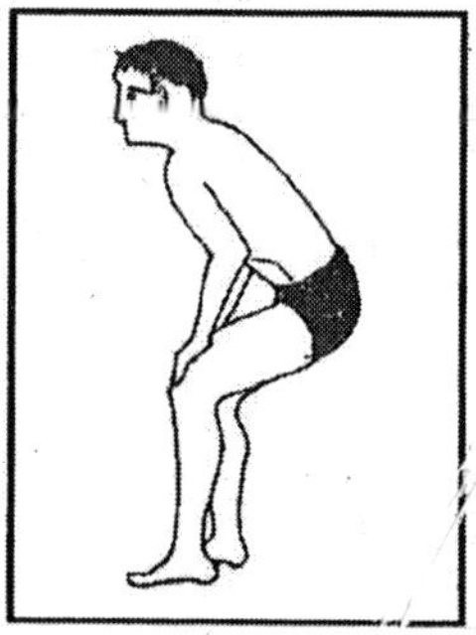

Fig. 89

Method: Sit in Padmasana or stand keeping the feet apart and place the hands on the knees. Keep the spine and neck straight. Eyes closed. No stress on any part of the body. Draw in a long breath. Lock in Mool Bandha. Draw out the breath slowly and relax the abdominal part. Contract the navel root towards the spine and loosen it. As long as external kumbhaka is maintained repeat it 10 to 100 times. Concentrate on Nabhi (centre of the belly or Manipur Chakra).

3. Plavini Pranayama:

Whenever the season changes the digestive power weakens. This pranayama develops the digestive power. It cures the histeria. It destroys the parasites of the abdomen. It expels all foul air from the stomach and cures all bilious disorders and abdominal ailments.

Method: Sit in meditative posture. Place the hands on the knees. Keep the body erect. Close the eyes keeping the mouth in a round shape, start sipping the air in the same manner in which water is sipped. Let the stomach be bloated with air. When the stomach is full with air, close the mouth for a few moments and hold the air inside. Keeping the tongue out and bending from the lumber region exhale the air completely out of the lungs. Repeat this process three times or more.

4. Ujjayi Pranayama:

This pranayama reduces the heat of the head and cures the cough, asthma, T.B. and other diseases of lungs. It kindles the gastric fire and activates the digestive system, the respiratory system and the nervous system. It makes the voice melodious and makes the heart strong, emotional balance is established. Throat diseases cured.

Method: Sit in any meditative posture or in any other comfortable pose. Keep the hands on the knees close the eyes, close the mouth. Contract the lower part of the tongue and the glottis and inhale in such a way that a sound resembling snoring is produced, of a mild and uniform pitch. Use light Uddiyan Bandha. Exhale slowly. Inhale from the both nostrils to the throat, from the throat to the heart. Then retain with comfort. While exhaling visualise the movement of the pran from heart to the throat, from throat to the nostrils. Exhale slowly. No sound is produced at this time of releasing the breath.

5. Bhramari Pranayama:

It increases blood circulation. Concentration of mind becomes easy. It gives immense joy. One who gets success in practising kumbhaka through Bhramari successfully enters the stage of samadhi. Tension is removed and anger turns into Divine love and calmness.

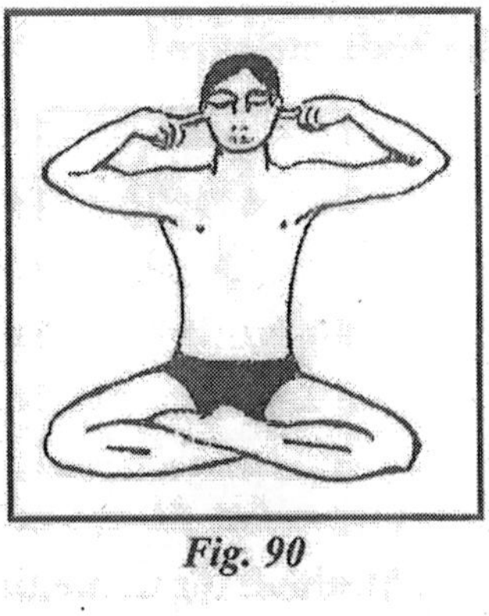

Fig. 90

Method: Sit in meditative or comfortable pose. Put the index fingers into ears. Close the eyes. Inhale deeply through the nostrils and exhale making a buzzing sound like a black bee. Listen to this mild himming sound. Repeat it five to ten times and then breathe in deeply and retain as long as you can with comfort. Then exhale slowly and resume normal breathing.

6. Bhastrika Pranayama:

This pranayama is performed rapidly and forcefully. It removes asthma and catarrh. It improves the condition of the throat. It gives the warmth to the body. It destroys the cough (mucus)

Method: There are four steps in this pranayama but here we give the last one. Sit in a meditative pose. Keep the hands on the knees. Close the eyes. Adopt the process of gold smith's bellows or like a panting dog. Inhalation and exhalation should be done rapidly and forcibly. To start with, practice ten inhalations and exhalations, then breathe in deeply, retain and exhale slowly. Do it three/four times observing Bandhas.

7. Chandra Bhedi Pranayama:

In our left nostril flows the cold air like the moon. To keep the body cool this pranayama is useful. It removes the fatigue and excess of heat in the body. High blood pressure becomes normal. It helps to have the mind calm. Many diseases caused by the excess bile in the body are cured.

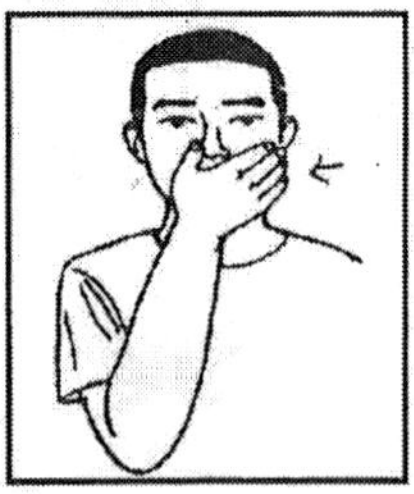

Fig. 91

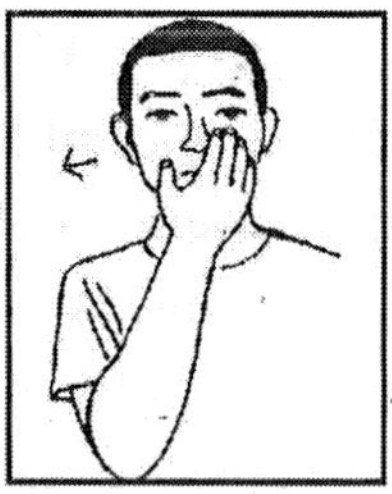

Fig. 92

Method: Sit in meditative pose. Put left hand on the left knee in gyanmudra. Close the right nostril with the help of right thumb. Inhale deeply through the left nostril. Retain the breath in antrik kumbhaka with the help of ring finger. Perform the three Bandhas, while doing kumbhaka. Exhale slowly through the right nostril. It is one round. Repeat five rounds and then rest. Every starting will be through left and exhalation through the right nostril.

8. Surya Bhedi Pranayama:

Suryabhedi pranayama increases heat in the body and removes the diseases caused by the disturbance of wind and phlegm in the body. It purifies the blood and enhances digestive power.

Method: The whole process is the same as in the Chandra Bhedi pranayama, but only one difference is that the inhalation is implemented through right nostril and the exhalation is done through left nostril every time. Repeat it 5 times in beginning and increase the rounds gradually.

9. Sheetali Pranayama:

It quenches the thirst and appeases hunger. It purifies the blood and destroys chronic dyspepsia and other diseases. This should be performed after Bhastrika pranayama. It removes the heat of body.

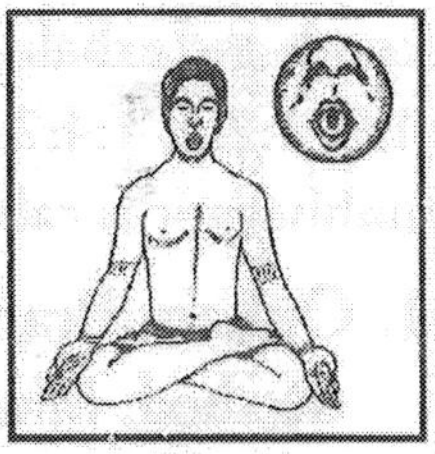

Fig. 93

Method: Sit in easy pose. The tongue should be pulled out and folded lengthwise like a tube. Draw in air through the mouth with a hissing sound and retain as long as you can with comfort, keeping the mouth closed. Then exhale slowly through both the nostrils. Repeat it six times.

10. Naadi Shodhan Pranayama:

It is called sukh purvak pranayama also. It aids digestion and improves the appetite, cleans the nasal passages and sinuses, purifies and enriches the blood stream. It has a calming and concentrating effect on the mind. This is an easier and less strenuous cleansing pranayama.

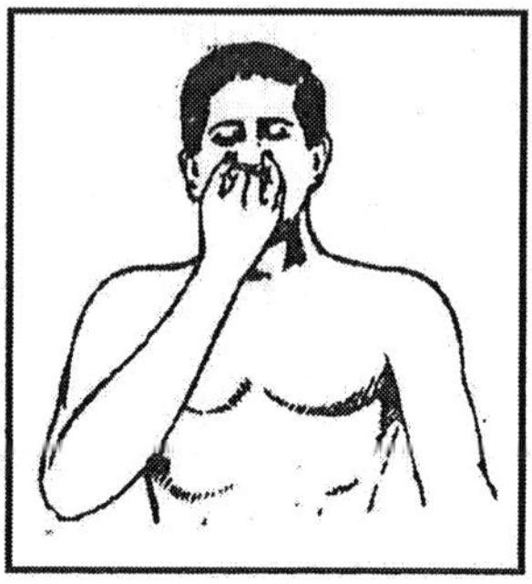

Fig. 94

Method: Sit in one of the meditative pose. Close the eyes. Put the left hand on the left knee. Close the right nostril with your right thumb. Inhale slowly and evenly through the left nostril, filling the lower part of the lungs, then the middle and upper lungs. There must be no forcing. Retain the pran for a few seconds, closing the left nostril with ring finger. It is the state of inner kumbhaka. Then release the right nostril and exhale slowly through it.

Now repeat the process, inhale through the right nostril, retain the pran and exhale through the left nostril. This is one round: The ratio should be 1: 4: 2. If you inhale only in 5 seconds retain 20 seconds and exhale in 10 seconds. The starting ratio should be 1:1:1, 1:1:2, 1:2:2, 1:4:2. Repeat the rounds 5 to 20 gradually. Without kumbhaka it is called Loma Anuloma pranayama.

11. Onkara Pranayama:

Method: Inhale through both nostrils and fill the lungs with air. Then produce the "O" sound of Om coming out from the navel. '000' at a mild, prolonged and harmonious pitch. When you are about to exhaust your breath close the lips and produce hum 'MMM', until the breath is completely let out. During this Pranayama concentrate on the Agya chakra. Practise this for 5 to 20 times to start with and then increase the rounds.

Benefits: It bestows peace of mind and illumination.

12. Kundalini Pranayama:

Method: While breathing in through the left nostril feel and visualise that the Kundalini Shakti is ascending from Mooladhara to Swadhisthana, from Swadhisthana to Manipur at the navel and soon until it reaches the Sahasrara in the crown of the head. Then makes a curve in the passage even like the handle of an umbrella and brings the energy in the space between the eyebrows at Agya chakra mentally reciting Om.

After retention breathe out through the right nostril visualising that the Kundalini retraces from Agya chakra to Sahasrara in the crown of the head, from Sahasrara again to Agya chakra from behind the head, from Agya chakra to Vishuddhi chakra, from Vishuddhi chakra at the throat to the centre in the heart, from heart to navel point from navel to Swadhisthana chakra and from Swadhisthana chakra to the Mooladhara at the anus.

Similarly breathe in through the right nostril, Retain and exhale through the left, visualising the same process. This constitutes one pranayama. Do it five times to start with and then gradually increase the number according to your capacity.

Benefits:

1. Awakens mystic kundalini.
2. Bestows various Psychic powers.

13. Pranayama for Relaxation:

Method: Lie down on your back on the Asana. Relax from the toes to the head or you may recline on your chair. Breathe in deeply without making any sound. Feel that you are filling yourself with energy, joy and peace.

Then exhale slowly and comfortably. Don't even think that you are exhaling. You may repeat "o–o–". While inhaling, and repeat "m–m" while exhaling. You may repeat any other mantra, half of it while inhaling and the other half while exhaling. Practice it fifteen minutes to half an hour to start with. Then increase the period.

Benefits:

1. It helps in complete relaxation.
2. It fills the body and mind with fresh energy.

14. Awakening of Sahasrara Chakra through Pranayama:

Method: Sit on a soft Asana near the wall. Inhale through both the nostrils in counting of 20 and exhale in five counting. Feeling that the breath is going to Sahasrara Chakra. Do it 40 times. Don't practice more than 10-15 minutes.

Benefits:

1. Sahasrara Chakra awakens.
2. It increases intellect.
3. It increases memory.
4. Freshness remains full day.
5. Eye-sight becomes better.
6. Mind becomes silent.
7. It increases magnetic power.
8. It prepares for Samadhi.

• • •

11

Pratyahara and Dharana

What is Pratyahara?

Pratyahara is a detaching of the mind from the sense-organs. It checks the outgoing powers of the mind and turns them inwards. It is a gathering in and integration of the previously scattered mental energies. In pratyahara one frees oneself from the objects of the sense-organs.

"When the senses have withdrawn from their objects and transmuted themselves into the modes of consciousness this withdrawal is called 'the **pratyahara**' —**Yoga Sutra (2/54)**

"An adept in yoga gives himself up to 'withdrawal' and stops the traffic of the senses with their objects which are word, sight, smelling, taste etc., to which they are invariably attached. He then makes his sense work for his consciousness and the ever-agitated senses are controlled. No yogi can achieve the aim of yoga without controlling the senses" **(Vishnu Purana)**

The external world is shut out in yoga meditation. The sense-organs (*gyanendrias*) themselves are merely the "middle man" between external world and consciousness. The eyes, for example, don't see in themselves but are merely the instrument of consciousness. The real organ of vision is in a nerve centre of the brain. A man may be asleep with his eyes open, performing the exercises in correctly and must bring the wayward attention back to its task. If mind is detached from the senses they become useless. Control of the senses is absolute one-pointedness of the mind. The senses are held in check by the Pratyahara.

Practice of Pratyahara

- Just as a tortoise draws in its limbs on all sides, so also the sadhaka, withdraws all his senses from the objects of the senses. Then his understanding is well-poised.
- "Be aware! Be alert. Be eternally vigilant. Cut all the desires with the sword of dispassion and the axe of discrimination. This is the true secret of self-restraint" says **Swami Shivananda.**
- Pratyahara becomes easy after the practice of ***pranayama.*** Pranayama should be performed with Om Mantra as Puraka, Kumbhaka and Rechaka.
- Remove these obstacles–unsteady asana, too much talking, too much walking, too much mixing with worldly people, intake of too much food, to much curiosity in others affairs.
- Perform yogasana with closed eyes. ***Shavasana*** is very helpful for Pratyahara. 20-30 minutes are sufficient.
- Practice recitations of–***Gayatri*** or ***Mritunjaya*** Mantra etc.,
- Concentrate on breathing or ***'Soham'*** Mantra with breathing.
- Perform Sanmukhimudra for 20-30 minutes.
- Perform ***Om 'Gunjan'*** sound loudly for 5-10 minutes in meditative pose with closed eyes.
- Hear the ***'Naad'*** with right ear for 30 minutes.
- Stop Sankalpa–Vikalpa in ***'maun'*** practice.

- 'Maun' can be performed for one day atleast in a week.
- Music is a tremendous means of pratyahara. Dhun *'ragas'* and classical music are helpful.
- Selfless service is also a good means for *'pratyahara'*.
- ***Trataka*** (inner/outer) is very useful. Trataka can be done on stars, moon, candle gazing, flowing water etc.
- Observance of silence, moderation in diet, patience, contentment, perseverance, tenacity, seclusion, right attitude, following yama-niyama, sakshi bhava, yogamudras, mental worship, keertan etc., are the aids for Pratyahara. Practise them.
- Yoganidra is the easiest and tremendous method for Pratyahara.

Benefits of Pratyahara:

- Pratyahara makes us introward.
- We can take sound sleep.
- Inner voice can be heard.
- Concentration becomes easy and strong.
- It increases will-power.
- Mind becomes silent and peaceful.
- We get success in meditation.
- We learn art of working.
- Our behaviour becomes controlled.
- Pratyahara increases inner spiritual strength.
- It controls emotional stress, worry and feeling of frustation.
- It controls the senses.

Concentration (Dharana)

What is Concentration?

"To maintain the mind fixed on one spot is called concentration." (Aphorisms of Patanjali 3/1).

Concentration is purely a mental process. It needs an inward turning of the mind. If you concentrate your mind on a point for 12 seconds, it is Dharana. Twelve such Dharanas will be a Dhyana (meditation). Twelve such Dhayanas will be a samadhi of (state of super consciousness).

Concentration is fixing the mind; meditation is allowing one idea to flow continuously. When by pratyahara the tyranny of the senses has been checked, it becomes easier for the mind energy to be focussed on one point. This action in yoga, is called concentration to an intense degree which can lead to psychic powers. Though these powers are not its absolute aim.

Dharana is another step on the path to self-realisation. Maharisi Patanjali says that yoga is restraining the mindstuff (chitta) from taking various forms (vrittis). The chitta be compared to the surface waters of a pool, and the vrittis are not thought waves that cross it. If we can still this flow of thoughts and hold the mind steady, then pure consciousness, our innerself, will be revealed and seen at the bottom of the pool.

Concentration is the key mastery of the mind and the emotions. Concentration is one of the chief secrets of success in every field—"*Genius is concentration*" said Schiller–Arjuna won Dropadi due to concentration. It is a famous story of Mahabharata in India. Concentration is the foundation of meditation. A piece of paper burns with the focussed sun rays for sometime. The blowpipe makes the hole in iron and due to focusing on a point. Like this power of concentration does a miracle in life.

Benefits of Concentration:

1. Concentration develops by Dharana by gazing consciously.
2. It develops good memory.
3. It increases awareness and deep observation power.
4. Concentration develops inner powers.
5. Confidence, particular thoughts and good nature is the result of concentration.
6. It purifies the 'Chitta' mind, intellect and ego (*Antahakarana*)
7. It develops will power also.
8. A Scientist gets new idea/invention due to concentration.

Obstacles in Concentration:

1. Lack of Confidence
2. Unsteady Nature
3. Short sitting
4. Irregularity in practice
5. To be much ambitions
6. Carelessness and laziness
7. Too much public relations
8. Scattered consciousness
9. Increasing 'Kleshas' of mind
10. An aimless life
11. Negative thoughts
12. Rajas and Tamas tendency
13. Dominant vayu element
14. Too much Sankalpa-vikalpa
15. Too much desires
16. Lack of patience
17. Too much physical exertion
18. Too much talking
19. Too much walking
20. Too much sexual indulgence
21. Too much anger
22. Illness

Aids to Concentration:

1. Cultivate attention, you will have good concentration.
2. Be cheerful always attention, than alone you can you have good concentration.
3. Be regular in your practice of concentration.

4. Celibacy, pranayama, reduction of desires and activities, dispassion, silence, seclusion, discipline of the senses, japa, control of anger, giving up reading novels and news papers, visiting cinemas, give up T.V. watching, are all aids to achieve concentration.
5. Japa and Keertana will develop concentration.
6. Stick to one centre when you concentrate.
7. Don't leave the practice even for a day. It is very difficult to rise up again.
8. Silence the bubbling thoughts calm the surging emotions.
9. Have 3 or 4 sittings, early morning 8 am, 4 pm and 8 p.m.
10. Devotee concentrate on the heart, Rajayogi on Trikuti (The seat of mind), vedantin on crown chakra.

Practice of Concentration

1. **Concentrate on a Concrete Form:** In the beginning concentrate on a flower, Lord Buddha, Sri Rama, Sri Krishna. Light of the heart, on the picture of any saint Hanuman or your Isht Devata.
2. You can concentrate on the tip of the nose, the navel, or the Mooladhara Chakra
3. **On Isht Devata:** Sit on any comfortable pose. Place a picture of your Isht Devata in front of you. Look at the picture with steady gaze. Then close your eyes and visualise the picture in the centre of your heart or in the space between the eye-brows.

   When the picture fades out in your mental vision, open the eyes and gaze at the picture again. Close your eyes after a few seconds and repeat the process.
4. Devotees of Lord Jesus can concentrate on the picture of Lord Jesus or on the cross, in the same manner as stated above or on Blessed Virgin Mary or idea of God.

5. **Black Dot (Trataka):** Concentrate on a black dot on the wall or a 8"×8" white sheet, a candle flame a bright star, the, moon, on the picture of Om or any other object pleasant to you. When you feel strain in your eyes, then close them for a minute and mentally visualise the object. When the mind runs, again and again bring it back to the object of your concentration. Concentration on moon is beneficial for emotional persons.

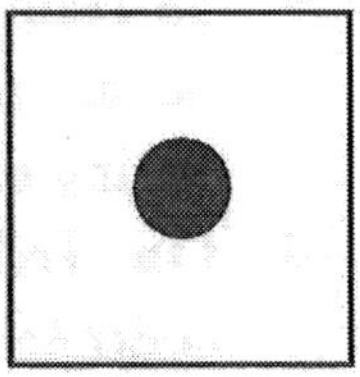

Fig. 95

6. **Divine Virtues:** Concentrate on any quality of God such as love, mercy, simplicity, kindness, truth, courage, generosity, honesty, humility, introspection, regularity, patience, purity, self-confidence, detachment etc.
7. **On Sounds:** Sit on any comfortable pose, eyes closed. Plug the ears with your index fingers or cotton plugs. Try to hear the inner astral sounds such as the music of the flute or violin, kettle drum, thunder, storm chiming the bells, blowing the conch, shell, humming the bees etc. Hear only one kind of sound. Withdraw the mental rays from other objects and merge them in the sound which you are trying to hear. You will get one pointedness of mind. The mind can be controlled easily because it is enchanted by sweet notes.
   - Concentrate on the tik-tik of a watch.
   - Sit by the river at a secluded spot. Concentrate your mind on the rushing sound of the river. You will hear the roaring 'Om'. This is very thrilling and inspiring.
8. **On mirror:** It is a sufi method. Place a mirror in front of you. Concentrate on the space between the eye-brows of your reflection in the mirror.

9. **So-Ham Mantra:** Concentrate on the breath in nostrils with Soham sound. There is '**So**' during inhalation and '**Ham**' during exhalation for 15 minutes at least.
10. **On Trikuti:** The mind can be easily controlled by concentrating on the Trikuti (between the eyebrows) Agya Chakra because it is the seat of the mind. When there is a deep concentration on trikuti you will experience great joy and spiritual intoxication. You will forget the body and the surroundings. All the pran will be taken up to your head.
11. **On Agyachakra (Shakshi Bhava):** Sit in any meditative pose. Eyes closed, concentrate on 'Agya Chakra'.Observe your mental condition, activities, thought etc. Don't clash with the thoughts. only observe. Your mind will be steady gradually. It will take one or two weeks. Increase the duration of your practice.

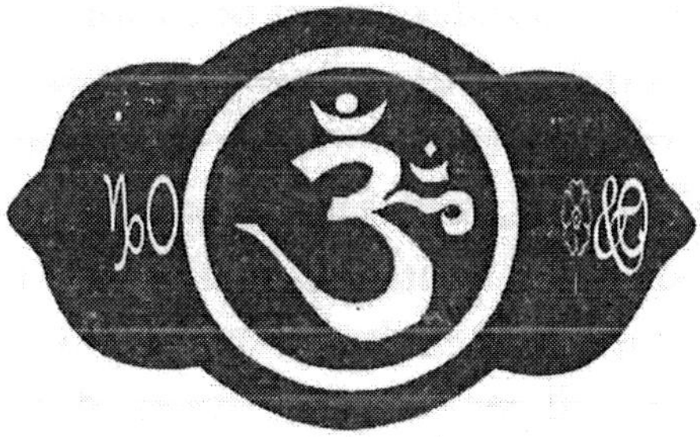

Fig. 96

There are many ideas for concentration such as. Aum Japa, Mental worship of Isht, control the mind forcely, selfless service, fasting, looking thoughts, creating thoughts disperse the thoughts, thoughtless state, concentration on earth, water, air, fire and akash tattvas.

Continuous and deep state of concentration becomes meditation.

• • •

12

Meditation

What is Meditation?

"Meditation is a process of leading the mind towards the subtler glories of creation, till the subtler field is transcended to get to the transcendental divine bliss."

—Maharishi Mahesh Yogi

"Meditation is the only royal road to the attainment of freedom. It is something mysterious, which reaches from earth to heaven, from error to truth, from darkness to light, from pain to bliss, from restlessness to body peace, from ignorance to knowledge, from morality to immorality."

—Swami Shivananda

'Meditation is a science of active silence.'

—Swami Vivekananda

"Meditation is an activity of the mental consciousness. It involves one part of the mind observing, analysing and dealing with the rest of the mind. Meditation can take many forms: concentrating single-pointedly on an internal object, trying to understand some personal problems, generating a joyful love for all humanity, praying to an object of devotion, or communicating with our wisdom. Its ulimate aim is to awaken a very subtle level of consciousness and to use it to discover reality, directly and intuitively."

—Kathleen McDonald

"Meditation is a mental device that limits stimulus input by directing attention to a single unchanging or repetitive stimulus. It has been observed to be an alter state of consciousness. Meditation can be used as a no cultic practice. It has been physiologically termed as 'wakeful, hypo-metabolic state.'

—Vashistha Samhita

"By meditation we correct the restless wandering of the mind and train it like an athlete to economise all its energies and fix them on the attainment of some desirable knowledge of self-discipline."

—Sri Aurobindo

Concentration and Meditation

Concentration is the sixth limb and meditation is the 7th limb of Astang yoga. Concentration helps to collect the mental rays from the diversified objects into a single forceful beam focussed upon a given/selected object. The intention of such concentration is to disentangle the mind from its involvement in the network of objects. Concentration can be on outer, inner and universal existence. Self-awareness is needed for concentration. Mind is dominant in concentration but a means to open to us the ***superconscience plans*** of our existence, concentration controls the mind.

Meditation is a deep and continuous concentration of focusing the mind on one thought wave, like unceasing flow of oil when poured from one pot to another. The mind flows towards God leaving behind all thoughts of the world. While stability, relaxation and concentration stages occur then awareness is added in meditation. Concentration is the base and meditation is the Bhavana (building). So meditation is to sit in silence home enjoying the company of our soul.

Concentration	Meditation
Concentration (One point) collection of energy on one. Point and establishes the consciousness on one object with control state of mind, waits for real knowledge in being introward. It is a trial.	Meditation is extention and deepness of concentration on one subject, thinking and getting peace with observation. Takes action with the entering object/wave/thought in the consciousness. It is a natural state in which we open towards the Divine. It is inner journey.

Meditation Poses

There are certain postures on which the meditation happens. These poses help in keeping the body and mind static and free from tension. The following are the main meditative poses.

1. Sukhasana (Easy Pose)
2. Siddhasana (Adept's Pose)
3. Padmasana (Lotus Pose)
4. Vajrasana (Lightning Pose)
5. Swastikasana
6. Gomukhasana

Why Meditation?

We should meditate regularly because the blessing of meditation are manifold:

1. Meditation is the most powerful, mental and nerve tonic.
2. 'Meditation kills all pains, sufferings and sorrows.
3. Mind becomes calm, serene and steady.
4. Meditation opens the door to intuitive knowledge and realms of eternal bliss.

5. Meditation is the key to unlock secrets of life.
6. It is the mystic Ladder which takes the meditator from earth to heaven.
7. Sadhaka will be able to face the battle of life with peace and spiritual strength.
8. The Divine energy forcedly flows in to the Sadhaka during meditation.
9. Meditation leads to self-realisation with burning aspiration.
10. Meditation increases intelligence significantly.
11. It provides safe and permanent solution to emotional and mental depression.
12. It increases the power of working and efficiency.
13. It improves memory and greater creative expression.
14. Meditation reduces negative emotions, such as fear, anger disappointment, miserliness, sexual passion, inferiority and superiority complex etc.
15. It keeps us in a relaxed state.
16. Meditation helps in lungs diseases, breathing problems, migraine headache, stomach disorders and blood pressure etc., and improves the physical health.
17. It improves the quality of sleep and significantly decreases the use of hard liquor and tobacco.
18. It develops the immune system.
19. In increases productivity.
20. It decreases drug abuse.
21. It enhances performance of work and play.
22. It fills with love sense of non-violence and truth.
23. Helps us in rediscovering the meaning of religion.
24. It reduces conflicts.
25. Is solves the riddle "Who am I."

26. It gives the power of discrimination.
27. It develops the willpower, the power of decision.
28. Meditation keeps the harmony of mind, body and sprit.
29. It is a very good source of personality development.
30. Meditation is useful for society, keeping the balance and good relations.
31. Sadhaka lives simple and sattvic life due to meditation.
32. Chetana becomes introward.
33. The consumption of oxygen is reduced due to deep and slow breathing.
34. The digestive system sets right.
35. The stormy tossing of thoughts is conquered.
36. The dualism of the consicousness, which expresses itself in the form of doubt, comes to an end and unity is gradually established.
37. Meditation is the best tool to purify the mind, chitta and ego.
38. Meditation helps us to know future events in our life, and guides about the Sadhana.
39. We get energy and Divine forces during the meditation.
40. Meditation is a means to offer and surrender ourselves to the Divine.
41. Through meditation subconscious releases hidden knowledge that allows better understanding.

Guidelines for Meditation

To gain full benefit following hints should be followed:

1. **The Place of Meditation:** It is very important factor to keep in mind. One should choose a quiet and peaceful corner or room of the home for meditation to abstain from disturbing surroundings and interference and to keep the sanctity of the practice.

2. **Time:** Morning and evening is the suitable time for meditation. Before going to bed is also useful for meditation. Braham Muhurta is charged with high spiritual forces and energy.
3. **Regularity and a fixed time is recommended:** Same place, same time, same method helps to settle the mind. Meditation easily occurs.
4. **Sitting Direction:** While meditating face should be in East/ North direction to get advantage of favourable magnetic and solar vibrations.
5. **Posture:** It is advisable to sit in a comfortable meditative pose. The beginner can sit in sukhasana but the advance Shadhaka should sit in Siddhasana/Padmasana keeping the spine erect and eyes closed.
6. **Asana:** Arrange white cotton bed sheet on four folded blanket.
7. **Empty Stomach:** Meditation should not be practised with a full stomach nor it should be done in hunger. It should be half full.
8. **Clothing:** During meditation one should wear according to the season, that does not constrain or produce a feeling of inhibition.
9. **Prepare the mind:** Prepare the mind for meditation by auto suggestion to calm down for a specific time, period, and detach from the external world and thought of past, present and future. Say like this—I am going to meet myself for half an hour. I am leaving the worldly thoughts out. I am going in to know who am I.
10. **Relax the body:** Relax the body. Think about one by one all parts of the body and imagine to relax.

11. **Regulate the breath:** Start with deep breathing or naadi-Shodhan pranayama, mind will be calm.
12. **Select one method:** Select one mantra, one chakra and one method, practise it sincerely.
13. **Starting time:** Begin the practice with 15 minutes and extend it to 45 minutes or 1 hour gradually.
14. **No Strain:** Meditation is an effortless movement of the mind and this should be done without straining the body/mind.
15. **Don't worry:** It does not matter how many times the mind runsaway. Bring the mind again and again on the line.
16. **Sit silently:** After the meditation. Sit silently don't destroy the bliss of meditation, starting any job just after the meditation.
17. **Meditate mindfully:** Be aware whole the day trying to concentrate your mind. Don't go in sleep during meditation.
18. **Control your emotions:** Try to control your emotions. Don't waste your time in gossipping.

Obstacles in Meditation

The main obstacles in meditation are sleep, tossing of mind, the rising up of latent desires, lack of celibacy (Brahamcharya,) spiritual pride, laziness, irregularity, disease, company of worldly people, over work, over eating, self assertive and Rajasic nature, are all obstacles.

- Conquer sleep through pranayama, asanas and light diet.
- Remove Vikshepa through Pranayama, Japa, Upasana, Trataka, etc.
- Destroy desires through dispassion, discrimination, study of books which treat of dispassion, enquiry, etc.
- Shunt out the company of worldly persons who always talk on sexual matters, money and worldly things.
- Obey the laws of health and hygiene.

Function and Purpose of Chakras

What is Chakra?

'Chakras' are psychic centres of activity of subtle, vital force termed Sukshma pran (Subtle pran). They are interrelated with the parasympathetic, sympathetic and autonomous nervous system, and thus the gross body is related to them.

'Chakra' is a sanskrit word that denotes circles, wheel and movement. Each chakra is a stage-by-stage play ground of desires. Energy moves through these chakras to produce different psychic changes produced by the endocrine glands whose secretions mix into the body's blood stream directly and instantaneously. Five tattvas (elements e.g. earth, water, fire, air and akash/ether) are the cause of these changes.

Our body is a mysterious creation of God. Kundalini shakti is sleeping in the root chakra. 7 chakras are the centres of Pran. They are said where the glands and the main nervous joints are described. We have five koshas. The main nerves Ida. Pingla and Sushumna channel are related to Kundalini. The chakras are the meeting place of the three naadis. Vajra and chitra are interior solar and lunar currents of sushumna. These all are in spine and in etheral body they resemble funnel shaped blossoms, each possessing different number of petals. Yantra , beeja mantra (sound), shakti, deity, Tattva and animal all essentials are symbolic and are shown in figures.

The chakras on the other hand act as a receivers transformers and distributors of the various forms of Pran. Chakras are the centres of power, vital force energy, Tattva, symbolic, full morality, source of spiritual progress controller of human body, health, knowledge and science. They move clockwise in men but anticlock-wise in women. There are different opinions about the numbers of chakras. Some says 88000 + 40 secondary some says 21 and some says 7 only.

Table of Chakras

Name of Chakra	Location	Colour	Petals	Alphabets	Elem-ents	Tattva Beeja	Glands	Prana	Loka Plane	Sense organ	Yantra Organ symbol	Work	Sen ses	Result of medi-tation
Mooladhar chakra (Basic) (1)	at the base of spine	Fiery Red	4	वं सं षं शं	Earth (Yellow)	LAM लं	Brahma Adrenal	Apana Vayu	Bhu	Nose	Square	Anua	Smell	Health Know-ledge
Swadhisthn chakra (Sex) (2)	Belov Navel	Orange (Sinduri)	6	बं भं मं यं रं लं	Water (Light Blue)	VAM वं	gonads		Bhu vah	Ton-gue	circle	geni tals	Taste	Peretry yoga siddhi
Manipur Knowled-- (plaxus) (3	Navel chakra	Yellow	10	डं ढं णं तं थं दं थं नं पं फं	Red	RAM Fire	Pancreas रं	Samana		Swah	eyes	Triangle	feet Legs	sight ge (vidhya) abiliry Stamina
Anahat chakra (Heart) (4)	Heatt	Green	12	क ख ग घ ङं चं छं जं झं ञं टं ठं	Air Smoky green	YAM यं	Thymus Adrenal	Prana Vayu	Maha	Skin	Hexag	hands	Touch	Wisdom Bhakti
Vishuddhi chakra (5)	Throat	Sky Red	16	अ आ इ ई उं ऊं ऋं लृं लॄं लॄं एं ऐं ओं औं अं अः	Akash Smoky purple	HAM हं	Thyroid Adrenal	Udana Vayu	Janah	ears	Crecent	mouth	hear-ing	Control on speech knowled-ge
Agya chakra (Master 3rd Eye) (6)	Between the eye brows	Indigo	2	हं क्षं	Maha Tattva	AUM ॐ	Pitui-tary	Vyana	Tapah	—	White	—	—	Soham siddhi Reali-sation
Sahasrar chakra (Crown) (7)	Top of the head	violet White	1000	अं क्षं	Beyond Tattva	— ॐ	Pineal	—	Satyam	—	—	—	—	Moksha complete Freedom

Description of the Chakras

1. Mooladhar Chakra:

It gives love, patience like mother 'Earth', harmony with earthly forces, energy, activity, creative, self-expression and leads to achieve consistency. It forms the vital foundation for all the higher chakras and is the source of the life force.

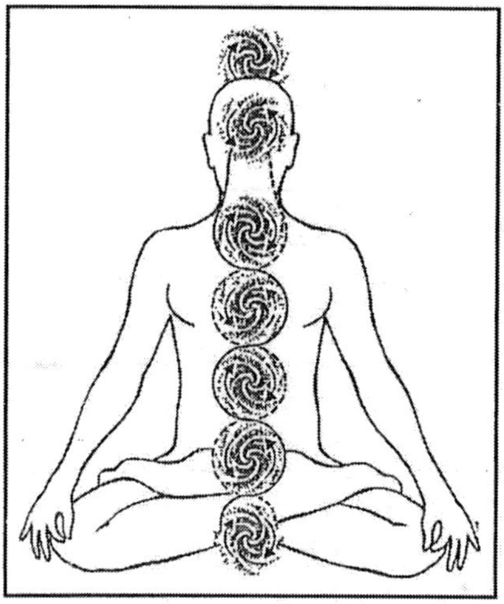

The direction of the chakras in men ←

The uninterrupted line spiralling up to the head represents *Pingla* while the dotted line symbolises ***Ida.***

Fig. 97

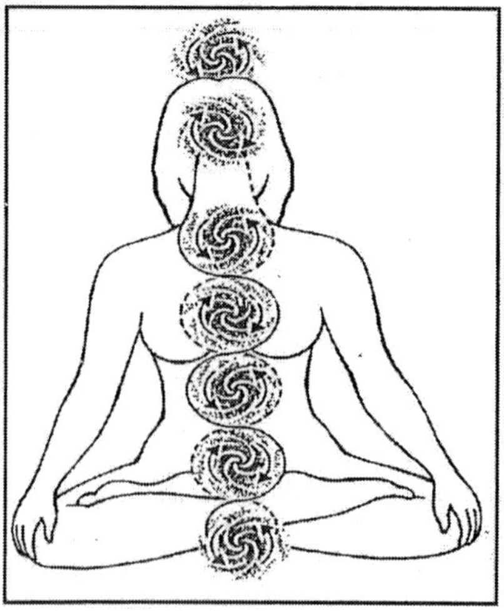

The direction of the chakras in women ←

The uninterrupted line spiralling up to the head represents ***Pingla*** or solar energy, while the dotted line symbolise ***Ida*** or lunar energy.

Fig. 98

A side view of the funnel-shaped chakras, their connection the main channel in the spine, and the way they radiate out from the physical body. ⟶

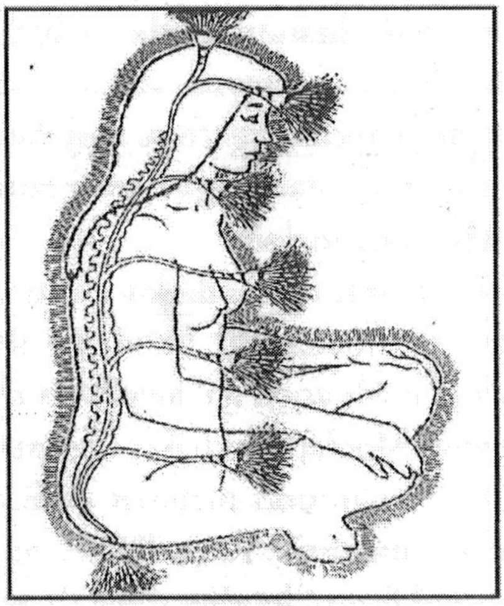

Fig. 99

Subtle body chakra centres of powers ⟶

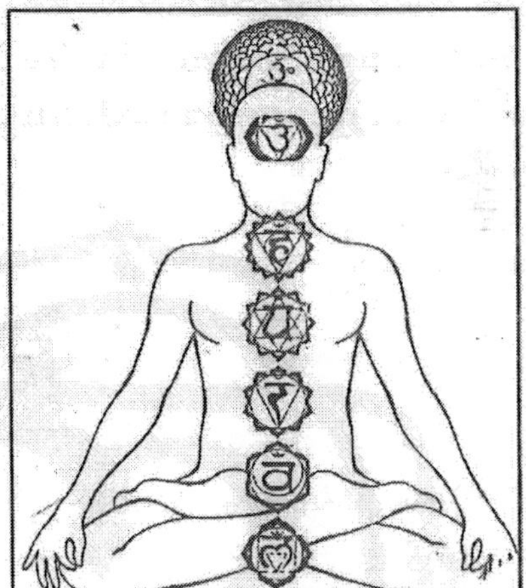

Fig. 100

Root chakra forms the centre of our system of subtle energy cycle. Moreover, it is the true seat of the collective unconscious. It maintains our inner balance.

Mooladhar chakra is related to all parts like spinal column, bones, teeth, nails, anus, rectum, colon, prostate gland, blood and building of cells, blood circulation and balancing of temperature of the body.

Due to meditation on the tip of the nose Sadhaka gets health, happiness, power of speech, victory, over earth element, awareness, freedom from disease, lightness, inspiration, vitality, vigour, stamina, security, an understanding of inner purity and softness in the voice and in the inner melody.

It is the seat of kundalini shakti. Activation of this chakra is necessary to awaken the kundalini shakti. Mantra, pranayama, Asanas and meditation are helpful in this matter.

If your Mooladhar chakra becomes imbalanced thoughts and action revolve around material possessions and security sensual indulgences and thrill. You will feel constipation, over weight, anger violence and fear of loosing some thing.

If your Mooladhar chakra is blocked, your physical constitution tends to weak. One keeps worrying has lack of stability and power to achieve. Swami Jyotirmayananda has given the detail description of the centres.

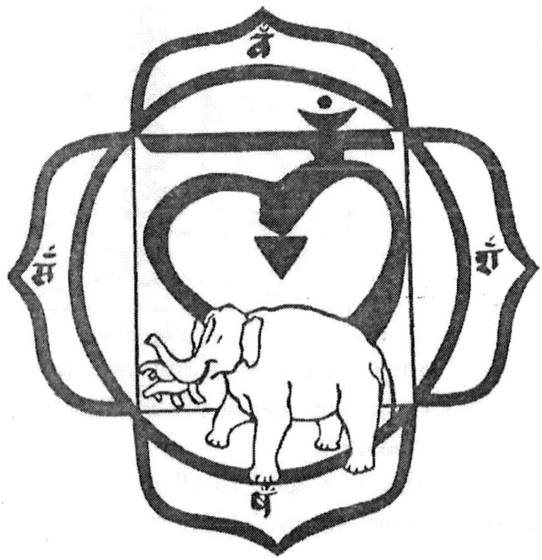

Fig. 101

2. Swadhisthan Chakra:

This is centre of unfiltered primordial emotions, the source of all biological life. It is the real seat of shakti, creative energy and sexual union. There is a natural flow of energy through body, mind and soul in it. Joy enthusiasm, action and creation, are its nature.

It controls pelvic girdle, reproductive organs, bladder, all liquids such as blood, lymph, gastric juice and sperm, gonard–ovaries prostate gland, testicles.

Fruit of meditation—Victory over the water, element, control of the senses, poetic skill, freedom from gross impurities such as passion, greed, hatred, egoism, pride, hypocrisy; reflecting the world, pure relationship with others, grace of Saraswati, knowledge, softness in nature (behaviour) wisdom is gained.

Its disharmonious function is awakening of sexual energies.

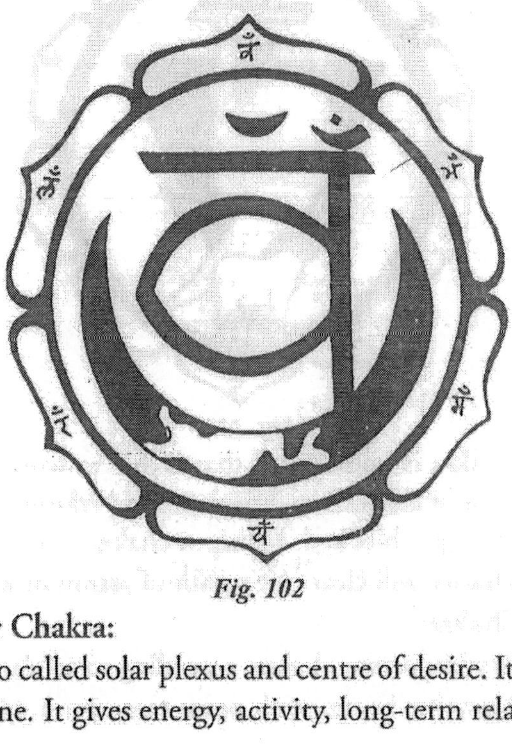

Fig. 102

3. Manipur Chakra:

It is also called solar plexus and centre of desire. It is the seat of spiritual plane. It gives energy, activity, long-term relations, full of joy, wisdom saving from danger and negativity, feeling of peace, inner harmony with yourself.

It is related to lower back, abdomen, digestive system, stomach, liver, spleen, gallbladder, autonomic nervous system. Pancreas, that balances fats and proteins.

The **fruit of the meditation** on this chakra are knowledge of the internal body, freedom from the ailments of the stomach, knowledge and power of human emotions, long and healthy life, egotism is lost, one develops the power to command and organise, control over speech and can express ideas very clearly, easiness in understanding the Naad.

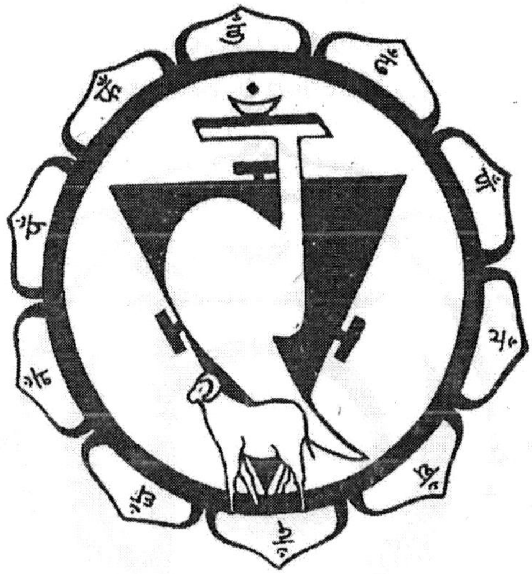

Fig. 103

If this chakra is imbalanced that is due to worry, castral ego, sensitiveness about cleanliness, miserness and taking of wine, drugs etc. the progress gets blocked. Manipur chakra is the centre of self-less service, charity will clear one's path of action or karma.

4. Anahat Chakra:

It is a very important chakra, according to Sri Aurobindo, it is the centre of psychic being, soul, pran, respiration, blood control.

It is a controller of all centres. It is the centre of Bhakti. There are three centres of mind, intellect and ego nearby. It is Hriday Guha.' Naad Brahm/is heard here. It is easy to meditate for ladies. It connects the three lower physical, emotional centres and higher mental and spiritual centres.

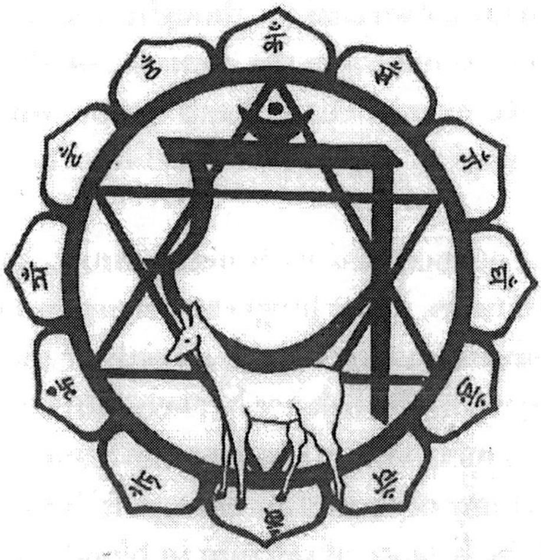

Fig. 104

The purpose of this chakra is to achieve perfect union through love, harmony, oneness and unity. Anger, despair for others, can be neutralised with deep love. Pain and illness are removed and spontaneous healing power is achieved.

This chakra is associated with heart, upper back, thorax, thoracic cavity, the lower area of the lungs and the skin also. The Thymus gland regulates growth and controls the lymphatic system. It stimulates and strengthens the immune system.

Fruit of Meditation: On this chakra gifts eloquence, poetic skill, victory over senses, hearing of mystic sounds, attainment of knowledge and psychic powers, mastery on language, mastery on own self, gaining wisdom and inner strength, male/female energy become balanced, life becomes source of inspiration for others, joy and parkaya pravesh (entering into the bodies of other persons) you love for love sake with no expectations from others.

5. Vishuddhi Chakra:

It is called throat chakra or communication centre, centre of human capacity of expression and inspiration. It is a bridge between lower chakras and the crown chakras, thoughts and feelings, impulses and reactions. It communicates the contents of all chakras to the external world. We express our joy and sorrow with words, arts, music, dance, thoughts, actions, and feelings. We maintain our freedom.

This chakra is associated with neck, throat, jaw, ears, voice, trachea, bronchial tubes, upper lungs esophagus, and arms. Thyroid gland plays an important role in the growth of the skeleton and inner organs. It governs the balance between physical and spiritual growth and via our metabolism, regulates the manner and the speed of the transformation of food into energy. It controls the iodine metabolism and the balance of calcium in blood and tissues.

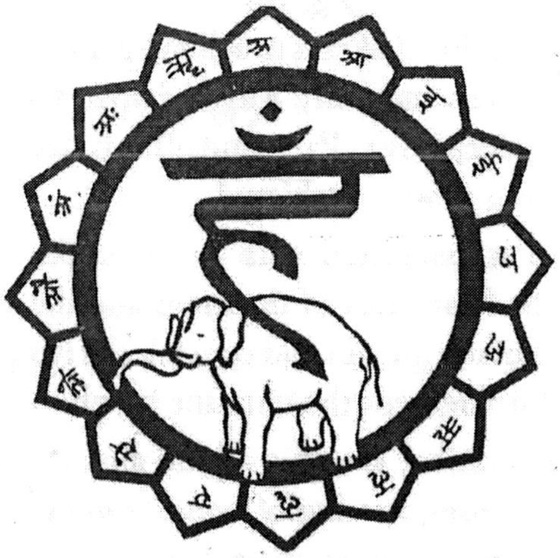

Fig. 105

By meditating on this chakra the sadhaka becomes poetic, wise, learned, peaceful, healthy, sorrowless, and leads a long life, possesses and controls on hunger and thirst, get purity and knowledge of past, present and future, serenity, melodious voice, command on speech understands the hidden message in dreams. He becomes a good teacher of spiritual science.

If throat-chakra is disturbed following diseases are seen—disorders of teeth, tongue, mouth, eye, nose, ears, arm and short constitution etc.

6. Agya Chakra (Ajna Chakra):

It is called medula plexus, Brow chakra, Third eye, The eye of wisdom, inner eye chakra, command chakra and guru chakra. Conscious perception of being take place through the 6th centre.

Fig. 106

- It is the seat of higher mental powers—intellectual capacity to distinguish our memory and our will.
- On the physical plane it is the highest centre of command for the central nervous system.
- It is the seat of attainment of consciousness.
- It creates new realities at the physical level and dissolved.
- We can sent out healing energy near and far.
- We gain intuition, clairvoyance or hypersensitive hearing or feeling. I had this siddhi.
- This expresses itself in an active mind and advanced intellectual skills.
- We can get reality through sleep or meditation.

- It is helpful in telepathy.
- Intuition and inner sight opens the way to all subtle planes of reality.

It is a spiritual gate to enter in subtle world. It is associated with face, eyes, ears, nose, sinuses, cerebellum, central nervous system, pituitary (master gland). This gland controls the other glands.

By meditating this chakra sadhaka attains the fruit of meditation of all the lower chakras. It controls the lower chakras. One attains Samadhi and destroys Karmas, sins, impurities and one enters the seventh door.

7. Sahasrar Chakra:

It is called crown chakra/vertex centre/ the 1,000 petaled lotus. The crown chakra is the seat of highest human perfection. It is connected with all the lower centres. It is the source and starting point for the manifestation of all other chakras/energies. It is the place where we feel at home, from here we once start our journey into life, and to this place we will return at the end of our development. Our personal energy field becomes one with the universe.

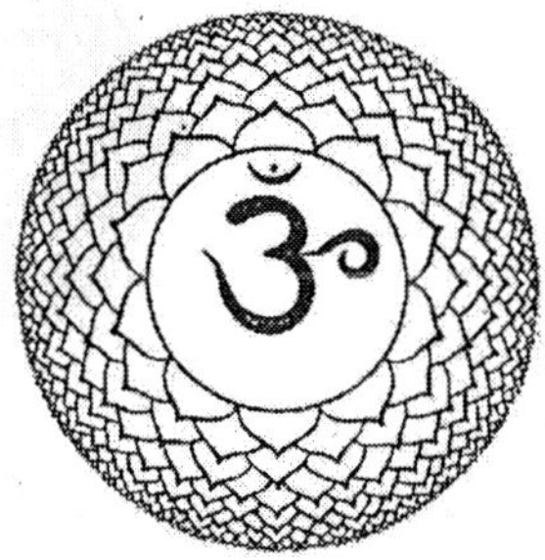

Fig. 107

The awareness given to us by the 7th chakra goes far beyond the knowledge conveyed by the 3rd eye chakra. Individual get ego transferred into universal ego. The realisation occurs. You translate the purpose of the Creator into action, in your behaviour.

The **fruit of meditation** on this chakra is immortality through highest samadhi, release from pain and rein carnation. Supreme bliss, knowledge of subtle forces, control on siddhis, complete peace, thoughtless state, forecasting the events, moksha and trikaladarshana etc.

How to Meditate

1. Simple Meditation

Method: Sit in padmasana/Sukhasana or Siddhasana. Put on the hands with Gyan Mudra on knees. Close the eyes. Relax the body from toes to head. Smile three times. Breathe ten times deeply and slowly. Make your mind complaintless. Say to yourself that I am going to meet myself.

Inhale and repeat 'om' rhythmically with sweet voice in ratio of 1:2. 21 times as an medium way 000 — mmmmmm. Do mental jap of om about 10 minutes.

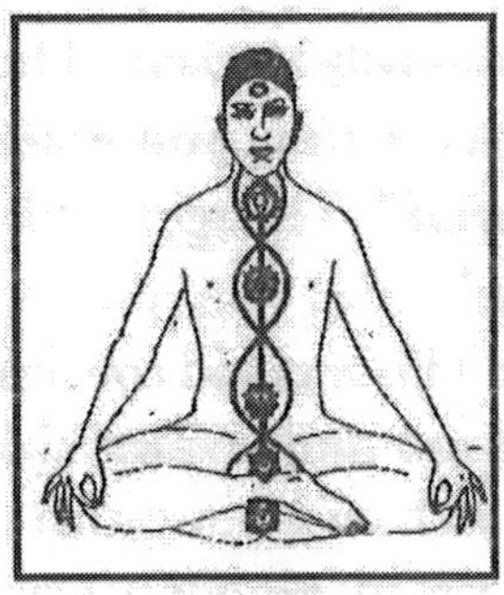

Fig. 108

Concentrate on breathing for 10 minutes. Observe the breath only. In the beginning 'So'—Ham mantra can help you to concentrate. Inhale with 'So' and exhale with '**Ham**'. Do it about 10 minutes.

'Who am I' think it over I am not body, I am not mind, I am not Pran. I am not intellect. I am above from these. I am a light and a soul.

Now, Pray for all. Pray your development, silently, you can concentrate on 'chakra' as well for better results.

Now, be silent for some time. Inhale and have a 'om' sound three times. Rub your hands and rub on face open your eyes sit for some time in this pose to prolong feeling of peace and bliss.

2. Watching the Thoughts: Sit in any meditative pose or on arm chair with the back resting. Watch the thoughts as they swarm about in the mind. Your mind is like a public place across which thoughts move in and out. A few attract your attention and remain for a longer time. Observe their play without identifying yourself with any of them. You will become aware that your consciousness— that is your mental self stands apart like a "silent witness" separate from the movement of the mental nature in you. On the other side this "witness consciousness", on the mental plane in you will help to stop the flow of thought waves in the mind.

Because you refuse to identify yourself with the thougths, their motion and insistence gradually weakens. The waves of the mental nature. Subside and after a time you enter into a state called *"quietude"* or *"quiet mind"*. Thoughts still occur, but they are subdued and don't disturb inner perceptions of the subject.

3. Mental Control: This method consists in creating a void in your mind. It is quicker and more radical than the above but also more difficult. You have to banish altogether all thoughts from the mind. As soon as one comes in, push it out or discard it right away, before it has time to settle clown. Not only should all reasonings be excluded in this way but all memories and associations too. Your mind enters gradually into the realm of "**quietude**".

4. Chakra Meditation:

1. Sit in a meditative pose with eyes closed. Concentrate on a Mooladhar chakra to be like a red rose opening to the morning sun. Concentrate on this chakra for 2-minutes.
2. Then imagine your sacral chakra (swadhisthan) to be like an orange coloured flower opening its bud, concentrate on it for 2 minutes.

3. Then imgine your solar plexus Manipur chakra to be like a yellow rose. Concentrate on it for 2 minutes.
4. Imagine your Heart chakra (Anahat) to be like a pink rose with a green stem opening up and emitting a white light concentrate on it as before.
5. Imagine your Throat Chakra (visuddhi) to be like a blue flower. Concentrate as before.
6. Concentrate on your Agya chakra (Third eye) to be like a dark blue coloured flower, concentrate as before.
7. Then imagine over your head a golden ball of light covering your crown chakra (sahasrar) and forehead with golden yellow light.

You can also visualise at each stage a white light like a cocoon around each chakra and imagine them to be protected from outside influence for additional benefits.

5. **Aura Meditation:** It is very interesting to note that the human aura changes drastically every hour depending on the individuals state of health, energy, levels, moods, thoughts and spiritual development.

Red in human aura denotes anger, fear, survival issues, material concerns and raw power.

Orange denotes sexuality, pleasure, warmth and passion.

Yellow denotes inspiration, intellectual activity, power of the mind and bright idea.

Green denotes balance, harmony, neutral influence, calmness and is a bridge between emotions, and higher reasons.

Bright Blue denotes healing, teaching ability, creativity, detachment and impulse to communicate to masses, all spiritual leaders have a very large band of bright blue colour and this has been proved by Dr. Kirlian. It is virtually not possible for ordinary humans to have such a stretch of Aura.

Indigo denotes intuition, psychic ability, spiritual protection. It bridges the two hemispheres of the brain.

Violete denotes wisdom, enlightenment and it bridges the physical mind with the higher mind.

Golden denotes brilliance, prosperity, spiritual radiance, higher creativity and the breath of the Divine.

Pink denotes purity and higher realms perception.

Method: Sit down as before, preferably in padmasana or sukhasana. As you concentrate, on your breathing, imagine you are sitting in meditation within a ball of white light floating in between. Concentrate for 2-3 minutes.

Then imagine yourself enveloped by a purple coloured flame and request the purple light mentally to cleanse your aura. Remain in this state of concentration for two minutes.

Then imagine yourself an emitting bright blue coloured band of aura. Imagine this band expanding continuously and radiating selfless love to all the people and objects around you. This will help you to develop unconditional love.

Then imagine yourself emitting a soothing pink coloured aura of light around you, and expand it as much as you can.

While imagining affirm in your mind's eye, "My aural vision brings the benefit of healing for myself and others and unconditional love to all creatures in this world."

6. Nirvikalpa Meditation: It is very effective meditation to make the mind thoughtless and nirvikalpa. Sit on soft asana near the wall. Close the eyes. Imagine our mind is a enlightened circle like a little plate. Think the thought as a black point of circle. Whenver any thought rises in your mind passout that thought through the circle. Until your mind remains enlightened you will be in the state of Nirvikalpa. In the beginning so many thoughts in the shape of black dots will come. Pass away those thoughts one by one. Mind will be thoughtless after some days meditation. You will get the Devine bliss. Meditate atleast 30 minutes daily.

7. **Meditation for Samadhi (Supper Consciousness):** Lie dow on the bed. Close the eyes with a cloth of blue colour. Relax the body. Imagine that this world is like a big blue star faraway. You are there. Bring in your chitta all the activities you do in your daily life as bathing, eating, working, reading, writing, worshipping, business etc. which you can do. You have forgotten your body. See your body as sakshsi Bhava only. Do it for half an hour for one year.

8. **Meditation on Senses:**

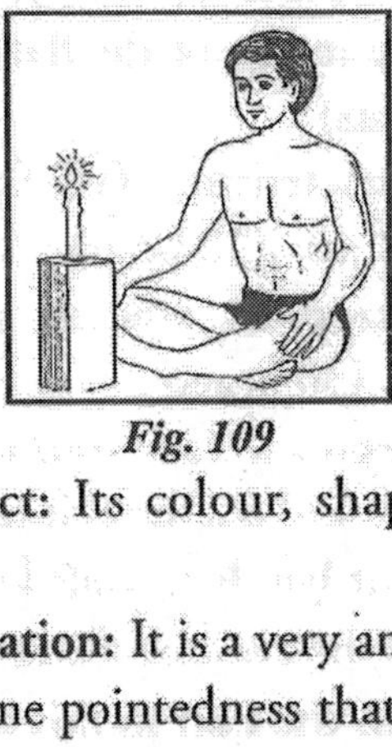

Fig. 109

(a) **On any object:** Its colour, shape, use, but not other thoughts.

(b) **Candle Meditation:** It is a very ancient and highly restful practice in the art of one pointedness that is, being able to direct your attention fully to one point and not allowing your mind to wander and waver.

This exercise is performed in two parts.

- **First:** Gazing steadily at the flame of a candle for approximately 2 minutes.
- **Second:** Placing your palms over closed eyes and attempting to retain the image of the flame for an additional 2 minutes.

- Before you start, your candle should be lit and placed about 3-5 feet from where you are. You should be seated in the usual padmasana posture. Then, fix your gaze steadily on the flame. Keep your eyelids in their natural position......Blink as you feel necessary.
- Observe now the subtle movements of the flame .... 30 beats = 30 seconds.
- Continue to observe the movements of the flame/...(30 beats)
- Now observe the various colours contained in the flame...(30 beats)
- Continue to observe the various colours contained within the flame....(30 beats)
- Now close your eyes and place your palms lightly over your lids...Retain the image of the flame and try to centre this image....(15 beats)
- Observe the characteristics of the flame now...the differences in form and colour...(30 beats)
- If the flame disappears, you can bring it back...simply by willing it back...(30 beats)
- As the image begins to fade continue to observe the subtle changes in form and colour as it fades....(30 beats)
- Now return your hands to your knees and open your eyes you may repeat the exercise if you wish.

9. Meditation with the Ear: In this sadhana we use our sense of sound and direct our entire attention upon ears. There are two forms of concentration-external and internal. For external concentration, choose a particular sound to listen. This can be a sound of nature such as the singing of a bird, a sound of water, a river, the ocean, the wind. When you find that your mind has wandered, you must bring it back again and again to the sound gently but firmly. Always give a mental order to the distracting thought which says in effect." I am busy now and I don't want to be disturbed."

A recorded music can be listened for five minutes. This music should be interesting. Sit in a cross legged position and lower your eyes. Listen very carefully to the music, there will be no thoughts at all. Attempt to make yourself an instruments through which the music may flow.

For internal hearing sit in a quiet place, either indoors or outdoors. Attempt to hear the sound within your own ear. There is a sound always present in you, this demands a complete withdrawal from the external world and is a fascinating challenge. If you can locate this internal sound which is similar to the sound made by the ocean waves striking the shore. Hold your attention upon this sound for three minutes.

Concentrate with the right ear for three to five minutes. It is tremendously, relaxing and refreshing. There are ten sounds like bee, shankh, ghanta, naad, flute and om. This is final. Practice as much as you can. Yoni Mudra can help to listen the naad.

10. Meditation with the Breath: This meditation is performed with your breathing. First, you must focus your full attention on the way in which you should be seated comfortably but firmly in the recommended posture, with your head straight and your eye lids partially lowered. Be relaxed---Now observe your breathing. It should be low breathing-that is, movement occurs only in the abdominal area. With each inhalation push the abdomen out slightly and mentally direct the air into the abdominal area. Do this easily ... without effort.

- Now attempt to slow the rhythm of your breathing.... (6 beats)
- Breathe as silently as possible....(6 beats)

- Now you are sitting correctly, breathing silently and slowly, and performing a slight abdominal movement each time you inhale...
- The next step is to establish a rhythm for your breathing. Count two pauses for inhaling .... two pauses exhaling and then rest without breathing for a count of two pauses.
- Now follow this rhythm. Begin to inhale: 1,2...exhale, 1,2...rest, 1,2....., inhale: 1,2...exhale, 1,2...rest, 1,2....., 2... Inhale, 2...exhale, 2... rest, continue this rhythm by your self: Inhale ; 2 .... exhale, 2... rest, 2.... Inhale, 2... exhale, 2... rest, 2..., Inhale, 2... exhale, 2... rest, 2...
- Now you must count your breath and focus your full attention on the counting. Each rest between breaths will count as one complete round... and you will count silently to 10 complete rounds. You must keep your attention concentrated or you will lose the count, Ready..Begin.
- Inhale, 2... exhale, 2...rest, 2... **Round 2:** Inhale, 2... exhale, 2...rest, 2...**Round 3:** Inhale, 2... exhale, 2...rest, 2... **Round 4:** Inhale, 2... exhale, 2...rest, 2... **Round 5: .... Round 6: .... Round 7: .... Round 8 : ....** Remember, don't allow your attention to wander **...Round 9: ....,Round 10:** ....rest.
- When you have finished 10 rounds, may continue this exercise for several more like units of 10 as you wish.

11. Meditation with the Voice: In this exercise, you meditate with the voice. You will be using a very ancient sanskrit syllable which has been chanted by millions of people throughout the centuries to experience a profound sense of peace.

The sound as you know about 'Om' is composed of two letters- 'O' and 'M'. To make the sound 'OM', hold the 'O' syllable for 5 beats -0-0-0-0-0. And then hold a resonant 'M' sound for 5 beats

...M-M-M-M-M.Then take a deep complete breath in 5 beats for the next repetiton.

The voice is medium-loud and steady. The sound should come from the abdomen, not the chest. The'M' sound is extremely and should be made to vibrate strongly.

- Sit in the recommended posture, Now perform the chanting...Hold your attention steadfastly on the sound of your own voice. Do not let your attention wander...
- Let us begin by taking a deep complete breath to a count of 5 beats, exhale completely. Breathe 1..2..3..4..5–0–0–0–0–0–M–M–M–M–M. Inhale 1..2..3..4..5–0–0–0–0–0–M–M–M–M–M.Deep complete, breath 1..2..3..4..5–0–0–0–0–0–M–M–M–M–M, and so forth.

  Throughout the chanting, hold your attention steadfastly on the sound of your voice. Do not allow your attention to wander.
- Begin once again, by taking a deep complete-breath for a count 5 beats exhale completely, then-00000-M-M-M-M-M. Inhale and repeat -00000-M-M-M-M-M Repeat each 'om' sound as many times as you wish.

• • •

13

Mind and its Control

What is Mind?

Mind is an internal organ in our body. It is one of the four important internal organs called, '**Antahkaran–Chatustaya**' viz, mind-intellect-chitt (memory)-ego. It serves as an instrument between the soul and the senses, as also between the soul and the brain in multifarious ways. Hence its importance can well be understood by the fact that all the activities of man in any shape of kind are always motivated by the mind. That is why in various upnishads, it has been stated quite clearly that whatever a man is, it is only because of his mind.

Mind is the only cause of a man's bondage of salvation. If the mind is engrossed in the sensual pleasures, then it results in bondage and if it is free from them, then the result is salvation.

In Sanskrit and Hindi, we call it 'mana' and its meaning is to know, to understand, to think or to ponder. If we go deep into its philosophy, man is called manushya or manava, because he thinks. So, in case a man does not think, he can't be called a man. That is what the etymological sense of the two words 'mind' and 'mana' when translated in Sanskrit/Hindi tells us. In Atharvveda, mind has been stated to be the cause of the cycle of births and deaths, but it is also the means which can help us to attain salvation.

The mind is situated in the head near the soul. It gets power from the soul. Some people say the nervous system is nothing but mind. Mental feeling is at the root of all our actions. 'Man is mind and mind is man' is a famous proverb.

Mind has control over the senses and without it the senses can do nothing. It has dual functions, i.e., on the one hand it directs the sense–both senses of knowledge and the senses of action, as also it conveys to the soul. So, it acts both ways inwards and outwards. Swami Dayananda says, "mind is that subtle matter in which there is only one thought comes at a time, though the speed of its thinking is so fast". Maharshi Vyasa says, "At the time of death, speech merges in the mind, all other subtle senses merge in the mind, mind merges in the 'pran' (breath system) and 'pran' merges in Tej (light) and Tej merges in the soul, which along with all, leaves the body."

Mind is composed of various subtle paramanus of matter and these paramanus have three kinds of properties, viz., Sat, Raj and Tam. The nature, capacity, power and working of the mind is bound to differ according to the ratio of 'Sat', 'Raj' and 'Tam'.

Controlling of Mind

To control the mind is very difficult because it thinks negatively and positively, speedily and on various aspects. Arjuna asks to Lord Krishna, "The mind is very agile and restless; it churns the man and it is very powerful. I consider to control the mind so difficult as to control the wind/air."

There are some points and techniques to control the mind. If we try to control the mind by regular practice we can get success.

1. Practice regularly to control the mind.
2. Develop the feeling non-attachment (vairagya).
3. Control the body to master or get perfection on one meditative asana.

4. Perform pranayama for about 15-20 minutes or more. If pran is still; mind will be still. This is the way to stop the wandering mind.
5. Mentally japa or loudly japa is helpful in controlling the mind choose one mantra and start chanting it.
6. Pratyahara, concentration and meditation techniques are very useful to control the mind.
7. Awareness is helpful to stop the negative thoughts, crowd of thoughts and to observe the thoughts.
8. Keep the mind busy in reading, writing, thinking, experimenting and observing the natural phenomenon.
9. The mind should always filled with noble thoughts. Reflect on noble things to study noble literature and to engage in the service of holy men.
10. Keep a distance from evil association, evil tendency; impure places, food, literature, sight, talk and surroundings.
11. We should always feel the Divine presence within and all round as guarding us from all evils, hostile forces and all our actions.
12. Be pure in your motives. Be honest and sincere in your efforts and behaviour. Think of other people's welfare and benefit, and keep away your selfish motives.
13. Believe that you are the master of your thoughts. Every individual has the power to control the mind.
14. Press the front corner of the tongue with teeth lightly or such as Khechari mudra is helpful in controlling the mind.
15. Think only one thing at a time and concentrate on a thought, the thought becomes true because our bodies, transform it into action. Recall the mind again and again.

16. Develop logical thinking to avoid the negative aspects. Don't follow the mind at once. Think and think seriously then take the decision and follow that strictly.
17. Discipline the mind to steady it by overcoming its vagrancy. The main causes of vagrancy are doubt, fear, restlessness, despondency, confusion and haste.
18. To over come doubting, develop self-confidence, superstition and delusion also give rise at the root of doubting nature.
19. Courage, toleration, perseverance in Sadhana, doing everything calmly and in a natural way remedies the habit of rashness.
20. Don't control the mind by force but control by reasoning.
21. Sit in meditation with this resolution that I will not give the chance to wander my mind.
22. If you feel the evil thought has come stop the breath at once. The wave of that thought will be cut at once.
23. Know the source of the coming thoughts.
24. Go in the deep of your mind. Peep into yourself. Search out your inner centre and set the mind there.
25. Sing the songs full of devotion.
26. Concentrate on light/sound which is interesting to you.
27. Purify your mind.
28. Concentrate on any chakra which you like most.
29. Bring back the mind from where it was slipped away.
30. Avoid gossipping and do social service.
31. Mind should be peaceful while you work. Maintain the peace in mind at any cost.
32. Be hopeful.

33. Pray sincerely for peace. You will feel peace in your body and mind.
34. Fix a target and try to achieve it strictly.

Special Yogasanas for Women

Ecpadasan; prarthanasan, Padmasan, Yasticasan, Parvatasan, Irikonasan, Garudasan, Hastpadungusthasan, Hastpadasan, Suptwajrasan, paryankasan, Ardhsarvangasan, Vipreetkarni, Bhujangasan, Shalbhasan, Halasan, Ustrasan, Makrasan (onbelly), Shavasan.

Qualities of a Yogi

If you want to be real yogi, you have to earn these virtues in life. Though Yama and Niyama are sufficient to live a yogic life these are some virtues but should be in yogi

1. Fearlessness
2. Wisdom
3. Knowledge
4. Charity
5. Purity of mind
6. Self-control
7. Concentration
8. Sacrifice
9. Austerity
10. Uprightness
11. Non-violence
12. Truth
13. Freedom from anger
14. Renunciation
15. Tranquility
16. Aversion of fault finding
17. Gentleness
18. Modesty
19. Forgiveness
20. Fortitude
21. Detachment
22. Desireless
23. Satisfaction
24. Simplicity
25. Awareness
26. Selfless service
27. Free from ego and hate

• • •

14

Purification of the Body

Role of Kriyas in Yoga

Our modern life is badly affected by pollution. Kriyas (the cleaning process) play the important role in purification of the body. Purification is first requirement of the body and mind to do the advance Sadhana of yoga. There are seven fold purposes of yoga hygiene.

1. **Purification of the body:** Kriyas are helpful to remove the impurities or mala shuddhi from the body. These kriyas bring down the body activity to a minimum level that facilitates the body working to go smoothly. Then body requires less oxygen to carry out its functions.
2. **Physical efficiency:** By the cleansing process the physical efficiency increases, Body and mind become light. The immunisation capacity develops. The body gets flexibility, free flow of respiration without any blockage.
3. **Longevity:** Sadhakas who know khechari mudra and do shuddhi kriyas daily, have achieved longevity. Pure body works more.
4. **Removal of Disease:** Shuddhi Kriyas help the individual to maintain good health but also cure the disease.

5. **Spiritual and Moral Elevation:** The aim of yoga hygiene is not only a mere acquisition of physical fitness but it aims at mental, moral and spiritual elevation which indeed depends upon the physical purity and well-being.
6. **Preparation for Asanas and Pranayamas:** Shuddhi kriyas are a precautionary system. They prepare us for asanas, pranayamas and meditation.
7. Kriyas are vital in influencing the imminent powers of body in developing specific immunity, capacity to resist and eradicate the offending factors and to help the body to recoup itself. Dhauti, Neti, Nauli, Basti, Trataka and Kapalbhati are the six Kriyas, practiced in empty stomach.
   - Cleansing materials for Dauti, Neti and Basti should be sterilized before and after the practice.
   - The water should be luke warm for Neti, Kunjal, Salt mixed luke warm water is used for Jal Neti.

Division of Shuddhi Kriyas

- Dhauti
  - (1) Antardhatui
    1. Vatasara
    2. Varisara (Shankh Prakshalana)
    3. Vahnisara
    4. Bahishkrita
  - (2) Dantadhatui
    1. Dantmula
    2. Jihvamula
    3. Karnar-andhra
    4. Kapalara-ndhra
  - (3) Hariddhatui
    1. Dand Dhauti
    2. Vamana Dhauti (Gajkarani/ Baghi)
    3. Vastra Dhauti
  - (4) Mulashodhan
    1. Ganesh Kriya
- Basti
  - Jala Basti
  - Shushk Basti
- Neti
  - Sutr Neti
  - Jal Neti
- Nauli
- Trataka
  - Bahya Trataka
  - Antah Trataka
- Kapalbhati
  - *Vatakrama
  - *Vyutkrama
  - *Shitkrama

1. **Cleansing by air:** Vatasara, shushka/sthoolbasti and kapalbhati.
2. **Cleansing by water:** Kunjal (vaman) varisara, (shankh-prashalana), Jalaneti, vyutkrama, and shitkrama, kapalbhati and jalabasti.
3. **Cleansing by friction or applicance:** Danda, dhuati, vastra duauti, sutraneti, dantmula, and Jihvamula.
4. **Cleansing by manipulating the organ:** Vahnisara, nauli, trataka and vatabasti.

Methods of Some Kriyas

- **Vatasara (Cleansing the intestine)**

Method: Draw in air slowly through the mouth forming it like the beak of a crow, move the abdomen and then slowly expel the air through the lower passage.

- **Bahiskrita (Cleansing the intestine and rectum)**

It is a difficult method of cleansing the air inside water, performed by retaining the air inside the intestine and passing it out through the lower passage and by cleansing the rectum with water. Now-a-days. Vatasana and Bahiskrita are not in practice.

- **Dant Dhauti Dantamula (Cleansing the teeth)**

Method: One should rub the root of the teeth with the extract of khadira plant bark (kattha) or with sand/soil until impurity is removed. Dataun of neem and Babool is better than paste and tooth brush.

- **Jihvamula (Cleansing the tongue)**

Method: Putting the first three finger into the throat, one should rub out the impurities and clean the root of the tongue slowly. Thus one can be free from diseases arising from phlegm.

- **Karnarandhra (Cleansing the ear)**

Method: One should rub the auditory canal by inserting the tip of the index finger into it. By constant practice an auditory sensation experienced.

- **Kapalarandhra (Cleansing the upper palate)**

Method: Every day, after waking from sleep, aftermeals and at the end of the day, one should rub the kapalarandhra (inner most part of the roof of the mouth) by reaching the thumb of the right hand there. The Nadi becomes purified and vision cleared.

- **Mulashodhana (Cleansing the anus)**

Method: Clean the rectum diligently with the stem of turmeric (plant), or with the middle finger and water again and again. This mulashodhana cures constipation and indigestion, gives radiant complexion and nourishment to body and stimulates the digestive organs.

Some Guidelines about Kriyas

1. Learn these kriyas by trained yoga teacher.
2. Kriyas generally practised in the morning in empty stomach (Dhauti, Basti, Neti, Shankha prakshalana) but the practices of kapalbhati, Trataka, Agnisar and Nauli can be done in the evening also.
3. It is advisable to learn the kriyas one-by-one as follows–Kapalbhati, jalaneti, rubber/sutra neti, vaman dhauti/kunjal kriya, Dand Dhauti and vastra dhauti.
4. To learn Nauli it will be the procedure–Uddiyana, Agnisar and Nauli.
5. After learning the Nauli perfectly then proceed to Basti.
6. Vastra Duati will be more effective if Nauli is performed in the final stage (after swallowing the cloth).

7. In advanced stage follow this order:
  - Vastra Dhauti (Nauli Chalana is to be performed in the, final stage), Danda Dhauti, Vamana dhauti or kunjal kriya, sutra/rubber neti, jala neti, and kapalbhati pranayama.
8. On the day of kriyas don't practice difficult Asanas as the body needs rest, but pranayama can be practised.
9. Shankha prakshalana and Basti should be practised separately. On different days, without combination of other kriyas like Dhauti as it may become heavy for the Sadhaka.
10. Trataka can be practised in regular during other your Sadhana.
11. Kapalbhati, Agnisar, Nauli, Trataka can be practised daily in the morning and evening.
12. Neti is generally advised once or twice in a week.
13. Dhauti, Basti and Shankha prakshalana should be done in every short period. They create very strong effect in the body. They are advised according to the need of the body, especially when the impurities to be removed from the body.

    Dhauti can be practised once or twice in a month. It can be practised once/twice in a week for the training period with Neti and Kapalbhati. It can be done continuously for few days in the morning to get rid of cold and asthma.
14. Generally, Basti is practised when the colon is to be cleansed. It is practised, once or twice in a month or even more if it is really required.
15. Shankha Prakshalana is generally advised once in three months or can be taken more than three as a short shankha

prakshalana because it cleanses the whole digestive system. February and October months are suitable for this kriya.

16. Kriyas should not be given the little children, mild practices like Neti, Kapalbhati and Trataka can be started as the age of 10 and according to the strength and capacity. Women during menses, persons, suffering from serious disorders are advised not to take these practices.

Techniques of Kriyas

There are eight main methods are used in yoga.

1. Neti Kriya

Neti is a cleansing process related to upper part of the respiratory system. It opens the nasal passage and to increase and sensitivity of the nasal. There are four types of Neti—

Types of Neti

Sutra (Rubber) Neti	Jala Neti
Ghrita Neti	Dugdha Neti

Neti Kriya cleanses the throat, eyes, teeth, ears and forehead. It helps in improving the memory.

(a) Sutra Neti

Required Material: Rubber Catheter No. 3 or 4/Sutra Neti, Warm water, Little towel, mustard oil.

Method: Take the Sutra Neti or a catheter. If using Sutra Neti drop it in water before use. If using a catheter put one drop of mustard oil on the thin part of the catheter. Catch the Neti with both hands with first two fingers and thumb check your nose from which side the air is flowing. Inhale from mouth and insert the Neti in the air flowing nostril and take out the end from mouth with the help of first two fingers of right hand. Wash the neti afterwards.

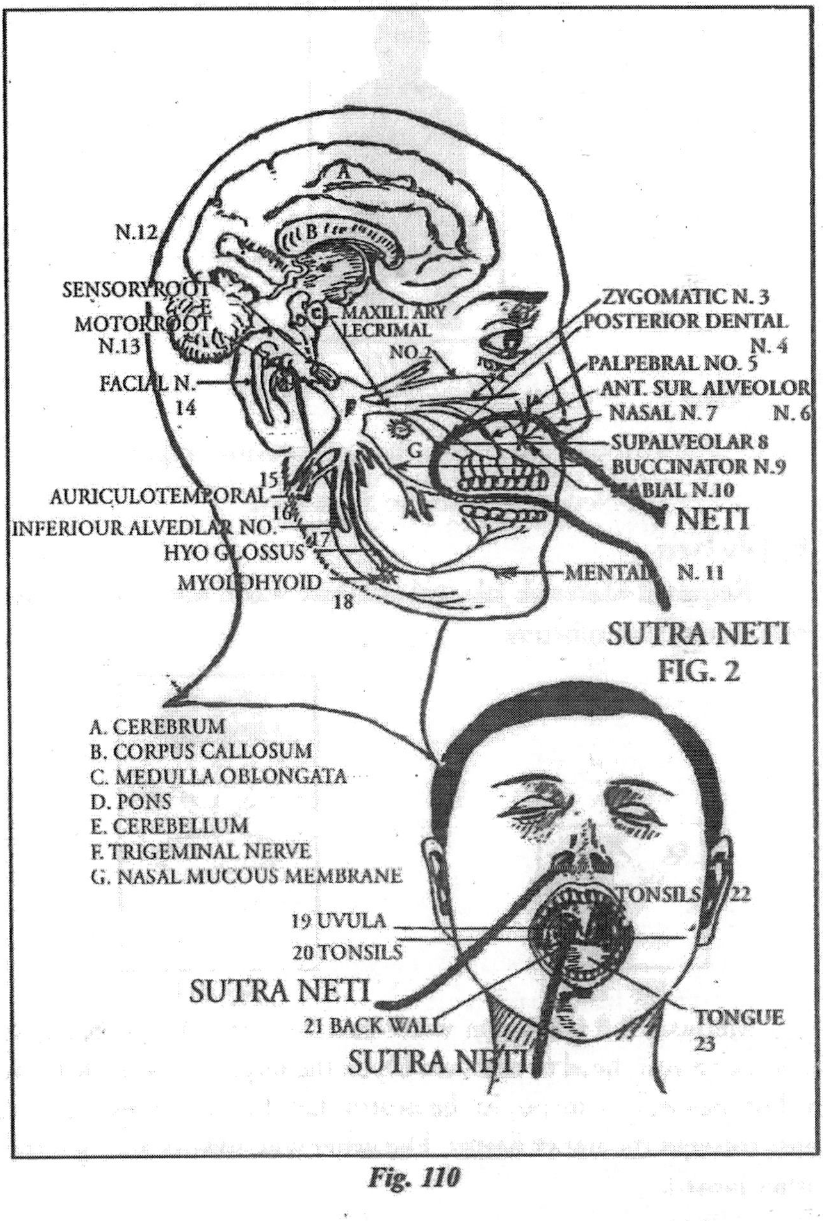
N.12
SENSORYROOT
MOTORROOT
N.13
FACIAL N.
14
MAXILLARY
LECRIMAL
NO.2
ZYGOMATIC N. 3
POSTERIOR DENTAL
N. 4
PALPEBRAL NO. 5
ANT. SUR. ALVEOLOR
NASAL N. 7
N. 6
SUPALVEOLAR 8
BUCCINATOR N.9
LABIAL N.10
NETI
15
AURICULOTEMPORAL
16
INFERIOUR ALVEDLAR NO.
17
HYO GLOSSUS
MYOLOHYOID
18
MENTAL
N. 11
SUTRA NETI
FIG. 2
A. CEREBRUM
B. CORPUS CALLOSUM
C. MEDULLA OBLONGATA
D. PONS
E. CEREBELLUM
F. TRIGEMINAL NERVE
G. NASAL MUCOUS MEMBRANE
TONSILS
22
19 UVULA
20 TONSILS
SUTRA NETI
21 BACK WALL
TONGUE
23
SUTRA NETI

Fig. 110

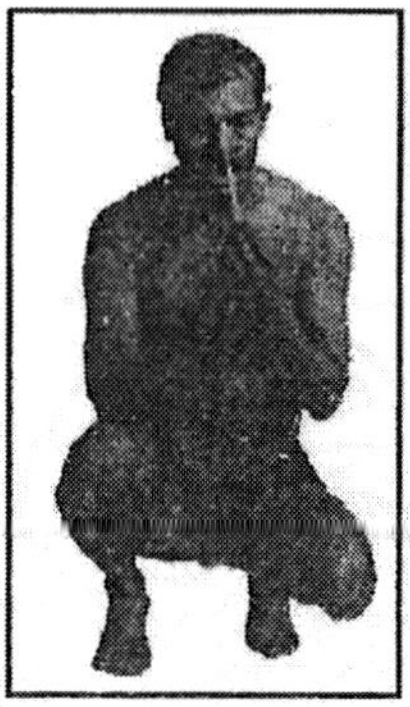

Fig. 111

Note:

1. Put a drop of ghee/oil in the nose previous night.
2. Do Jala Neti afterwards the Sutra Neti.

(b) Jala Neti

Required Material: Jala neti pot, luke warm water, in summer fresh water. Salt, tub/tray.

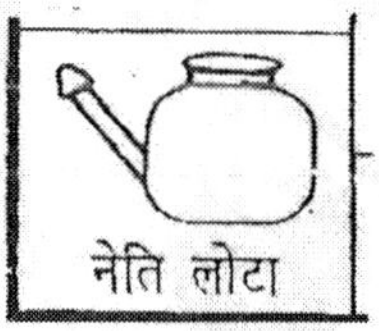

Fig. 112

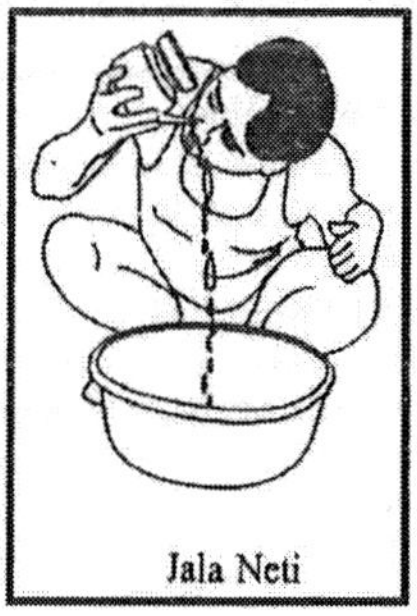

Fig. 113

Method: Fill lukewarm water in a Neti pot. Mix a little salt in it. Bend your head to one side. Open the mouth and inhale from it. Put the beak of the pot in the nostril. Let the water flow into the nose through the upper nastril. The water will flowout through the other nostril.

Initially, this may give an unpleasant experience repeat it on the other side. You can drink the water through the nose.

Note:

1. Do Kapalbhati pranayama after Jala Neti.
2. In summer and in case of nose bleeding fresh water is used for Jala Neti.
3. Do it after Shankha Prakshalana also.

(c) Ghrit Neti

Required Material: Pure ghee of cow, dropper/spoon/cotton a little pot for ghee and towel.

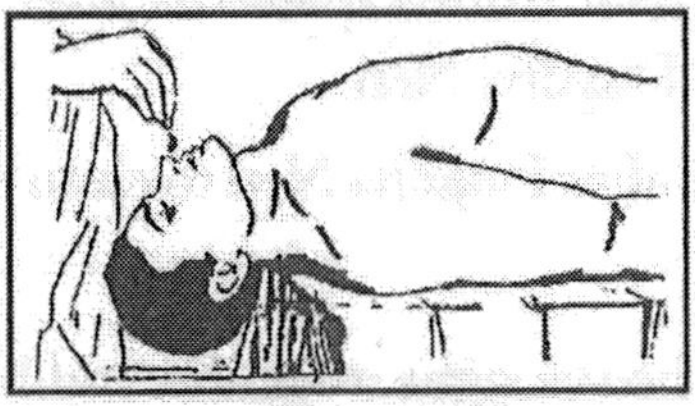

Fig. 114

Method: This kriya should be practised at before night or before sutra neti or jala neti. Lie flat on a table or floor fill the dropper with lukewarm ghee and drop some drops in both nostrils. Cover the face from the towel. You can do this kriya with the help of spoon or cotton.

Benefits:

1. It looses the phlegm and it comes out easily.
2. It destroys the dryness of the inner nose.
3. It removes oldest headache, weakness of the brain.
4. Ghrit Neti increases the memory and thought power.
5. It helps in good sleep.

(d) Dugdha Neti (Milk Neti)

Required Material: Jala Neti Pot, Fresh Cow Milk, towel.

Method: Sit in kagasana like Jala Neti put the beak of milk Neti pot in the right nostril by the right hand. Close the other nostril with the thumb or index finger. Keep the head backward. Drink equal milk through the both nostrils.

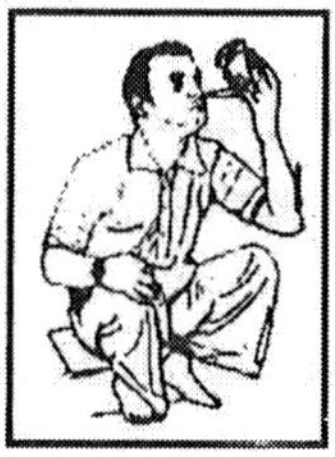

Fig. 115

Note:

1. Clean the brain from kapalbhati after the Jala Neti then practise the Dugdha Neti.
2. Do Jala Neti after Dugdha Neti to clean the nose and throat.

Benefits:

- It removes the eye sight weakness and hair disorders.
- Dugdha Neti increases the memory and mental power.

2. Dhauti

Dhauti means to wash. There are five types of Dhauti.

Types of Dhauti

(a) Vaman Dhauti (Kunjal Kriya)

(b) Vahinisara (Agnisar)

(c) Vatasara Dhauti (Kaki Mudra)

(d) Vastra Dhauti

(e) Danda Dhauti

(a) Vaman Dhauti (Kunjal Kriya)

It is also called Gaja karni. To cleanse the stomach and food pipe, have good practice of drinking lukewarm water and vomiting it. It removes extra acid, bile and cough and helps in poor digestion, bile diseases, acidity, asthma etc.

Required Material: Glass, mug, bucket, towel, 2 litre luke warm water, salt is used at first time, tub etc.

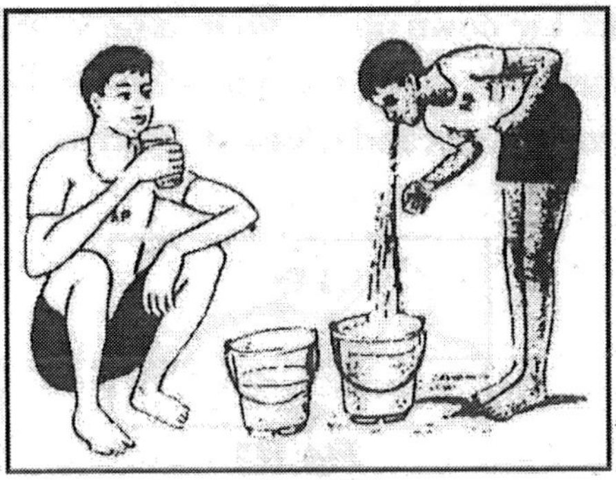

Fig. 116

Method: Sit in Kagasana. Drink five or six glasses water quickly. Keep both hands on the knees, stand up at 90° angle, bending forward and tickle your little tongue to induce vomiting with the three fingers of right hand, along with the left hand on the stomach Use the uddiyan bandha, water will come out gushing. Do it until the stomach is empty. Stand straight, wash your mouth and face, perform Kapalbhati and lie in shavasana for 5 minutes.

Note:

- Drink water quickly. Put some water in the mouth when you change the glass.
- Keep first three fingers of right hand in the mouth until the stomach is empty.
- Keep forward bending until the kunjal kriya gets finished.
- If you have high blood pressure do it with fresh water without any force and salt.
- Perform Kapalbhati when you stand straight after Kunjal Kriya

(b) Vahnisara (Agnisara) Dhauti

It is called Agnisara kriya. It can be performed in three ways. First in lying position, secondly in padmasana or vajrasana and thirdly in standing position.

(i) **Method:** Lie down on the floor upon your back, bend your knees so that the heels touch the buttocks. Do Bahya Kumbhaka draw the navel to the back and release it. Practise it about a hundred times.

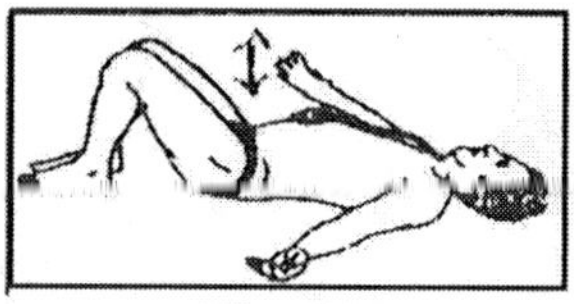

Fig. 117

(ii) **Method (in padmasana):** Sit in padmasana. Put your palms on the knees, Exhale do the Bahya Kumbhaka and draw the navel to the back and release it. Do as much as you can. Increase the number upto a hundred strokes.

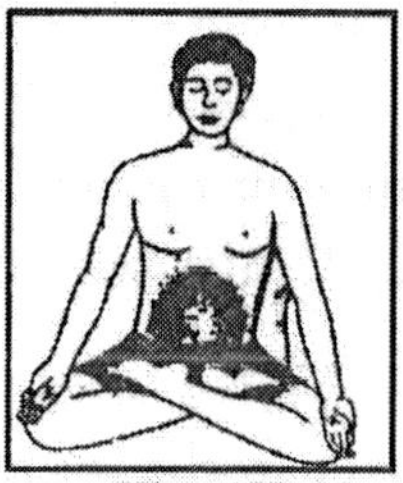

Fig. 118

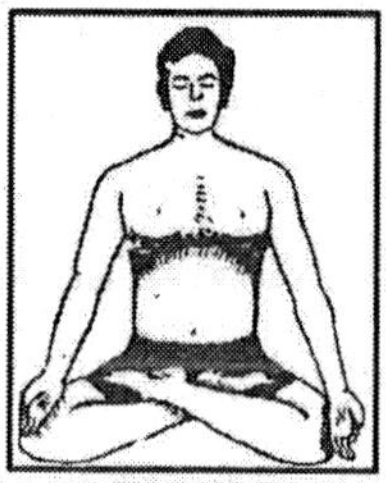

Fig. 118 A

(iii) **Method (in standing position):** Stand up keeping the legs apart. Put your hands on your knees. Exhale and perform the Bahya Kumbhaka draw the navel to the back and release it. Do as much as you can. Increase the strocks upto hundred times.

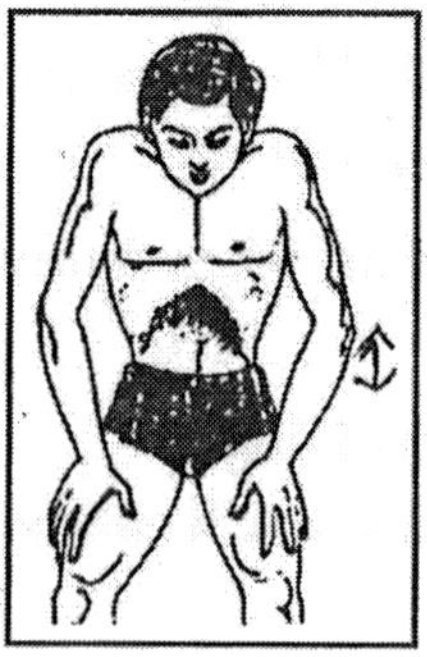

Fig. 119

Benefits:

- Abdominal obesity is reduced.
- Cures constipation.
- Increases appetite.
- Apana pran is equally strengthened by this kriya, and it helps in the proper excretion.

(c) Vatasara Dhauti

By contracting the lips, draw air through slowly until stomach is filled. Then practise this kriya and expel the air through the nostrils. This is also known as Kaki Mudra/Kaki Pranayama.

This purifies all the Nadis or the astral tubes. The body is rendered light and healthy. It controls the gas/vata.

(d) Vastra Duati

Required Material: Vastra Dauti (cloth), water/milk, towel, salt pot, cloth 3" (breädth) × 22'5" m length a finely woven cotton fabric like muslin (malmal) is suitable. The borders of the cloth are delicately but neatly stitched, soft white muslin is ideal.

Method: Vastra Dhauti can be practised either in standing or sitting position (utakatasana). Sit in a comfortable position. Keep the pot with Dhauti and water pot 2' apart.

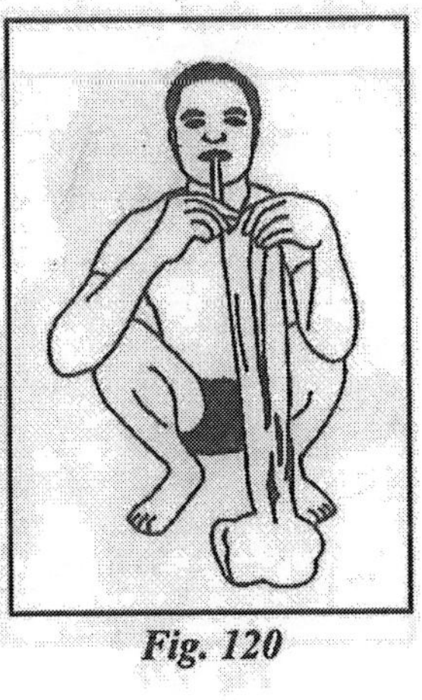

Fig. 120

- Take one end of the cloth while the rest of the cloth is immersed in water/milk. Fold (2-3 small folds) forward and backward and place it at he root of the tongue.
- The fold should b: in such a way that it opens up easily as it moves down the pharynx. Drink a sip of water/milk and swallow the cloth, continue swallowing like food.
- If there is sensation, stop for some time till the spasm gets relieved, then continue swallowing.
- Swallow till 1-2 feet is left out side. Perform Nauli chalana. So that the cloth rubs and massages the stomach.
- Stop the practice and pull out the cloth carefully using the fingers, Don't use force.
- Time duration for the whole practice should not exceed more than 20-25 minutes.

(e) Danda Dhauti

It is a cleansing process related to digestive system which effects more on respiratory system. Danda means a stalk (tube) which cleans the upper part of the digestive system with the help of a stalk. In modern method a rubber tube about 90 cm long and 0.5 cm bore is used in the place of plantain or turmeric stalk since the rubber tube can be used many times after sterilisation.

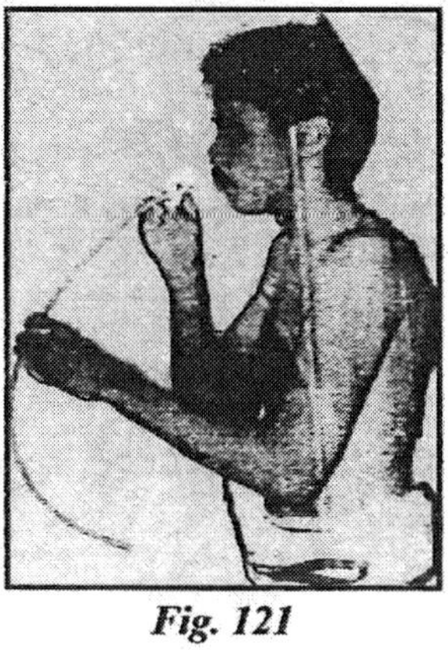

Fig. 121

Required Material: Danda/rubber tube, salt, water (Luke warm), bucket, towel.

Method: Drink 4-5 glasses of luke warm salt water. Slowly and gently introduce the small end of the tube into the mouth.

Move and push the tube slightly inside and simultaneously perform swallowing action so that the tube enters into the food pipe and not inside the wind pipe. One third portion of the tube is left out side the mouth.

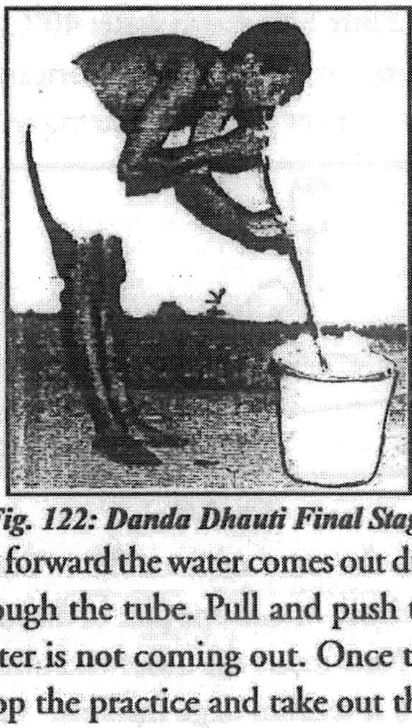

Fig. 122: Danda Dhauti Final Stage

Slightly bend forward the water comes out due to Siphon action automatically through the tube. Pull and push tube smoothly and carefully if the water is not coming out. Once the water has come out completely stop the practice and take out the tube gently.

Note:

1. Check the tube there should not be any cut or damage in the tube.
2. Sterilisation of the rubber is important before and after the practice.
3. Clean and lukewarm water should be prepared.

4. In the beginning practise Danda Dhauti without drinking water.

3. Basti (Enema)

It is a method of cleansing the rectum and colon. It is a cleansing process related to lower part of the abdomen, large intestine. Nauli and Naulichalana kriya and Uddiyana Bandha is necessary to know.

Required Material: (1) smooth tube of around 6" made of metal or rubber. (2) 2 litre luke warm water 40°C (should be boiled fully). (3) salt, (4) tub, (5) towel (6) oil (lubricant/soap)(7) enema pot with tube and nozzles or pumping enema set.

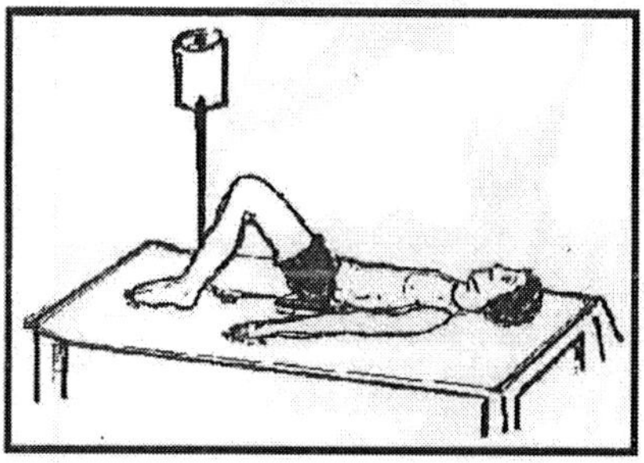

Fig. 123

(i) Method: Lie flat on a table or floor. Take a long smooth tube smeared well with oil. Attach one part of the tube to a container/ bucket full of water. Now insert the other end into your anus. Keep inserting the tube till it reaches large intestine. Hold the water for some time. After removing the tube and go for latrine after Nauli Chalana.

(ii) Method: Sit for latrine in kagasana. Insert the nozzle into the rectum upto large intestine. Put in the another end of the pump enema set. Have pumping slowly. Hold the water inside for some time. Remove the tube and sit for latring after Nauli Chalana.

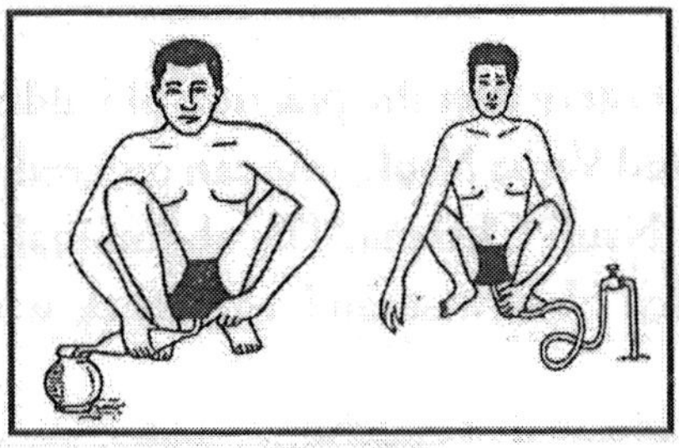

Fig. 124

Benefits:

1. Basti/Enema removes constipation, enhances digestive power and strengthens the body.
2. The brain functions get altered. Mind becomes stable emotional reactions to external stimuli are altered.

4. Nauli Kriya

What is Nauli?

It is a vigorous exercise for the stomach. It removes dyspepsia, liver troubles, enlargement of spleen and various diseases of the stomach. It bestows radiant health.

"Rapidly move the abdomen from side to side is called lauliki or Nauli. This destroys all diseases and increases the heat of the body."

—Gherand Samhita

Previous Practice

Uddiyana Bandha (The raising of the Diaphragm) in padmasana, vajrasana, utakatasana, tadagi mudra (in lying position) and viparita karani.

Types of Nauli

1. Madhyama (central aspects) Nauli
2. Dakshina Nauli
3. Vama Nauli

Naulichalana

Having got mastery over the practices of Uddiyana Madhyama Nauli, Dakshina and Vama Nauli, one can proceed to the final stage of Nauli called as Nauli Chalana. The abdominal rectimuscles are isolated then rolled clockwise and anti-clock-wise several times continuously.

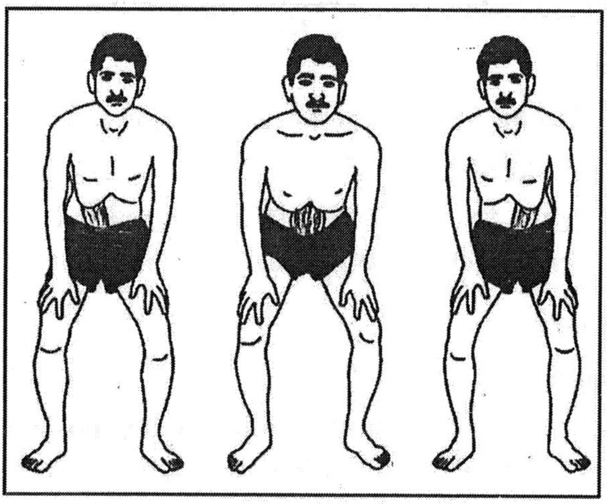

Fig. 125

Nauli Chalana Clockwise

Uddiyan Bandha
↓
Madhyama Nauli → Dakshina Nauli → Uddiyan → Vama Nauli → Madhyama

Nauli Chalana Anti-Clockwise

Uddiyan Bandha
↓
Madhyama Nauli → Vama Nauli → Uddiyan → Dakshina Nauli → Madhyama

Method: Expel air forcefully through the mouth and draw the navel to the back. This is Uddiyan Bandha. Release the tube like muscles in the middle pressing on the thighs. Release the tube like muscles to the left side. It is called Vama Nauli, when the muscles come to the right side it is called Dakshina Nauli. After good practice of Nauli start Nauli Chalana clock wise and anti clockwise.

5. Kapalbhati Pranayama

Kapalbhati means shining the forehead or skull. This is purificatory exercise.

Method: Sit in padmasana/siddhasana or any other comfortable meditative pose. Perform quick exhalation with very short inhalation perform Bahya kumbhaka and exhale the pran again and again. Don't try to take the breath. Push back and forth the obdominal muscles.

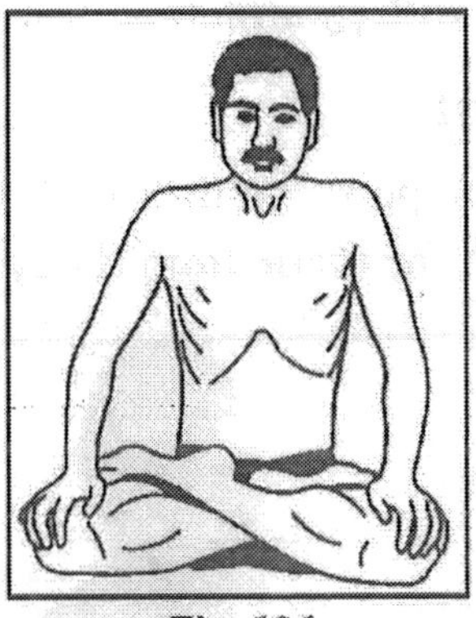

Fig. 126

To start with the practice ten expulsions followed by deep inhalation. Then retain as long as you can comfortably do so then exhale slowly. Take normal breaths.

Benefits of Kapalbhati Pranayama:

1. Helps to clean the sinus and respiratory passages.
2. Stimulates and tones up the abdominal muscles.
3. Fills more oxygen into the lungs.
4. Enlightens the brain and purifies the mind.
5. It is very beneficial for lungs and heart.
6. Improves blood circulation.
7. Destroys Kapha accumulated in wind pipe.

8. It strengthens liver, intestines, pancreas, digestive system and removes the fatness.

6. Trataka

Gazing or staring at a particular point is called Trataka. This is a cleansing process prectised with the help of eyes. There are two types of Trataka–(1) Bahya Trataka (2) Antar Trataka

Required Material: Candle/Deepak, Matchstic, ghee/oil, Trataka Yantra/picture of god or guru.

Previous Practice: Any meditative Asana like—padmasana, vajrasana, swastikasana, with gyanmudra,

Method of Bahya Trataka

Sit in any meditative pose. Put the candle flame at the level of eyes and at a distance of one metre from the eyes.

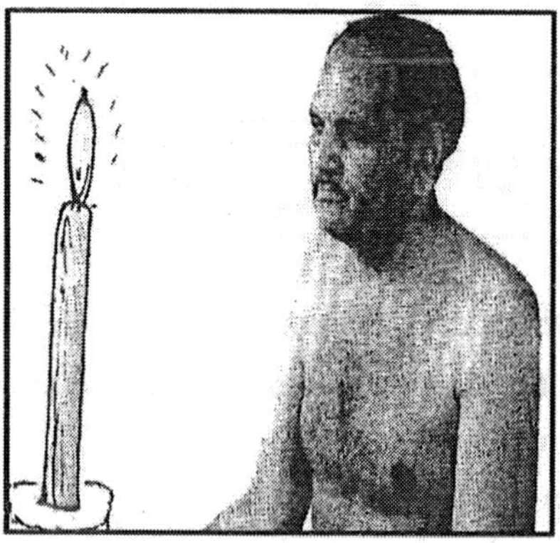

Fig. 127: Bahya Trataka

Close the eyes and relax the body completely. Open the eyes and gaze continuously at the flame. Don't blink your eyelids or move the eye balls. Without effort try to gaze the flame. Tears may come out. Maximum length of practice is for 2 to 3 minutes and then gently close the eyes. Practice should be comfortable.

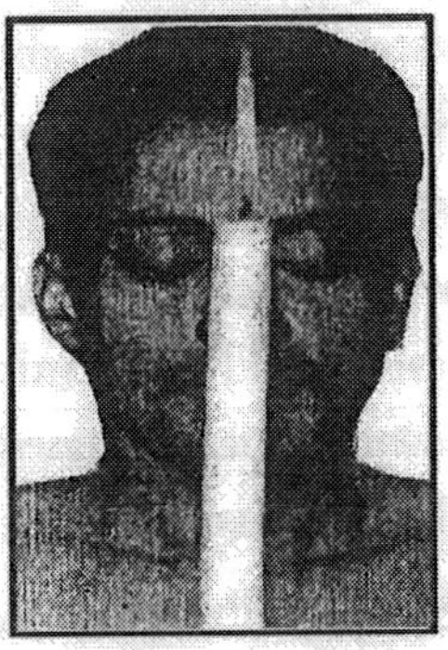

Fig. 128: Antar Trataka

Practice Bahya Trataka for few rounds carefully, close the eyes gently and gaze the after image of the same object inside. Repeat again and again. Have palming for 2 minutes and wash eyes with cold water in the end.

7. Shankh Prakshalana

It is a cleansing process related to digestive system with salty water. Shankh means conch, our small intestine is compared to spring (or) conch.

Required Material: Lukewarm water about 20 glasses, salt, glass, towel, bucket, mug, lemon.

Previous Practice: Practice of Nauli Chalana, viprita karani, tadasan. Tiryaka tadasana, katichakrasana, tiryak bhajuangasana and udarakarshana, vakrasana, mayurasana.

A light semi-liquid diet in the evening and night on the previous day of shankha prakshalana.

Method: Boil 20 glasses of water. Add 4 tea spoon common salt and one lemon juice. Let it cool. Sit on kagasana and drink two glasses of this water. Perform 5 yogasanas or more five times.

After consuming 6 glasses of water go for natural call. Now take two glasses of sline water. Repeat the above asanas. And again answer the naturals call. Repeat the process.

By and by, 16 to 20 glasses of water have to be taken in the end, you must be able to pass clear water without any colour or particles of dirt. Stop the process. Take 5 minutes rest. Do Kunjal drinking 3 to 4 glasses of water. Lie in shavasana for half an hour. Eat Khichari mixed with 100 grams ghee.

Five main Yogasanas of Shankh Prakshalana

1. **Tadasana:** Stand erect keeping your feet together. Raise your heels up and arms over head with the palms upward. Inhale and stretch as much as you can. Return slowly the heels to the ground. Repeat upward stretch five times.

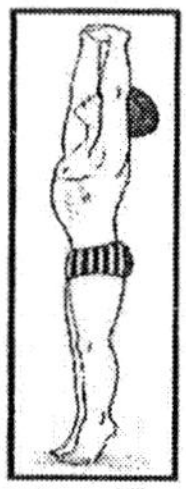

Fig. 129

2. **Tiryaka Tadasana:** Take tadasana position. Keeping the feet apart. Bend to the right and then to the left with antrik kumbhaka. The movement is from the waist. Bend five times each on either side, Breathe deeply.

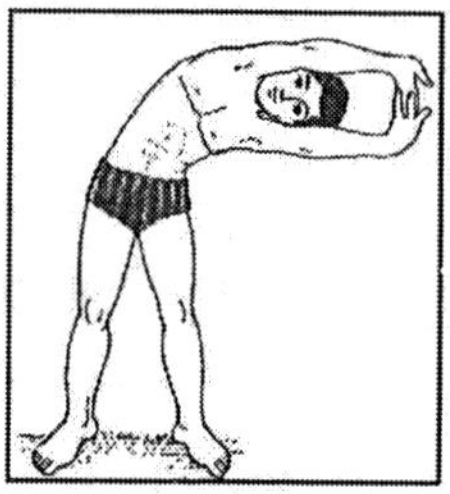

Fig. 130

3. **Katichakrasana:** Stand erect with your feet about one foot apart. Stretch the arms infront of your face. Stretch the arms side ways at shoulder level twist the upper part of the right shoulder and wrapping the right arm around the trunk in a smooth motion. Repeat on the opposite side. Five times each on either side.

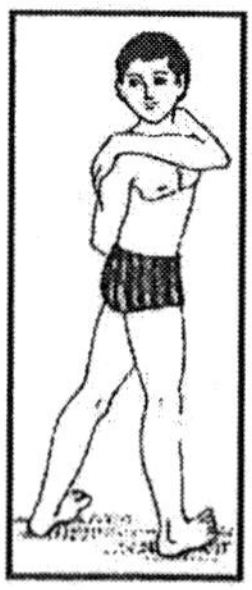

Fig. 131

4. **Tiryaka Bhujangasana:** Take the final position of basic Bhujangasana, twist the upper portion of the trunk and head to one side and gaze at the heels. Do it in opposite side of the body. Repeat it five times for each side.

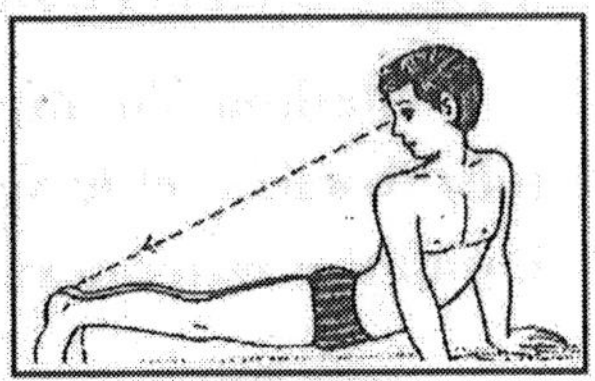

Fig. 132

5. **Udarakarshana:** Sit in utkatasana (squatting pose) with hands on the knees. Bend the left knee to the ground while turning the trunk to the right. Look behind the body keeping the hands on the knees. Return to starting position. Repeat the same procedure, twisting the body in the opposite direction five times each on either side.

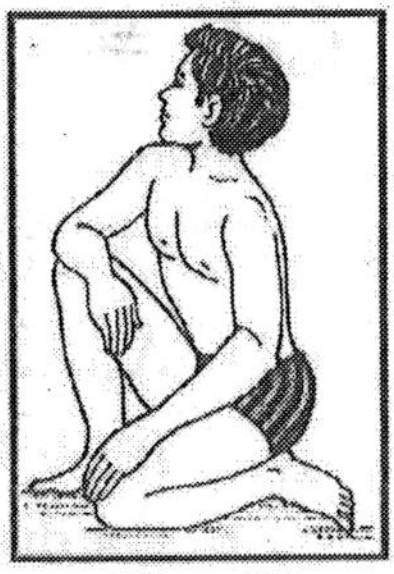

Fig. 133

Note: Don't take bath after shankha prakshalana.

- Eat Khichari of moong, rice and 100 gms ghee during the day.
- Don't drink water and sleep for about three hours, after the shankh prakshana.
- Don't take milk, curd, sweet, pickle for three days.
- Don't do this exercise if you have H.B.P. or heart problem.
- Do it after 6 months when the season is changed.
- This kriya removes kidney stones, constipation, acidity, gas and other digestive disorders.

8. Ushapana

Drinking water in the early morning is called ushapana. It is very useful to keep the mind cool and eyes sharp. It removes the constipation. This ushapana is performed through nose or mouth.

Required Material: Copper pot full of water, tulsi leaves/bael leaves/Rudrakhsa seed.

Method: Put drinking water in copper pot you can add some tulsi (bacil)/bael leaves or one Rudraksh seed in it before night. Drink this water next morning.

Take drinking water in a glass. Put this water under the nose and inhale. Slowly and gently till you feel the water in the throat. Now, you have to go on drinking the water in usual way. Drink it daily.

Note:

- Don't inhale forcefully.
- Agnisara andUdarakarshana are performed after the usha pana, the bowels becomes clear.
- For diabetes use bael leaves in water.
- Use Rudraksha seed in low blood pressure.
- For removing the worms of stomach use tulsi in the water.
- It protects from many diseases.
- Don't drink water in hiccup, wound and pneumonia.
- Don't take the water just after drinking castor oil.

• • •

15

Purification of Consciousness

Consciousness (chetana) has four parts as-mind, Wisdom, Chitta and Ego is called Antahkarana. Without the purification of consciousness the man's ultimate goal—self-realisation can't be achieved. The seeds of diseases are in the mind. Mind controls the senses. Wisdom justifies the decision. Chitta is the tap recorder of our karmas good or bad of the wordly life. Ego is the base of our life to implement our desires.

There are some yogic techniques that are needed to purify the consciousness:

1. Yama and Niyama:

According to patanjali's 'yoga-sutra' yama, is particularly very useful for society. There are five forms of Yama-Ahimsa, Truth, Non-Stealing, Celibacy and Non-greediness. Niyama is a personaly code of conduct. There are five forms of Niyama-cleanliness, content-ment, austerity, study of scriptures and surreder to the lord. The Yama and Niyama are the basic fundamentals of Raja yoga. They purify the body, mind and chitta. Ego is also reduced. Daily introspection is necessary. Maintaining a diary is also helpful.

2. Pranayama:

'Pran' is the connecting link between body and mind. If you control pran and sexenergy you can control the mind, conscious mind and sub-conscious mind (Chitta) through pranayama. Pranayama makes the mind pure and silent. It helps in purifying the chitta. Body and mind are cleaned by deep breathing, Anulom-vilom, nadi-shodhan, Bhramari; chandra bhedi and Suryabhedi Pranayama. Negative thoughts turn into positive thoughts. Pran is the life force cleansing the subtle body, mind and thoughts. Mind becomes fit for meditation by pranayama. Pranayama helps to awake the kundalini shakti.

3. Meditation:

Meditation is the spiritual practice of purification of consciousness. It cuts our old sanskaras (karmas) form subconsciuos mind. We stop the new impurities coming into the mind through meditation. We reduce our desires and ego. Abhyasa and vairagya are helpful in meditation. We must mind some points to prepare for meditation, as–static body, faith and confidence, surrender to God, steadiness of the mind, regularity, non-interruption, one pointed dhyan, fixed time, fixed place, fixed asana, fixed Isht, fixed mantra. Meditaion can be done on music, mental Jap, virtues, thought creation, thoughtless state, breathing, chakra, om sound etc prove helpful.

4. Desireless Action/Service:

Desireless service purifies the consciousness easily. We should perform some work for others without self interest with love for their welfare and without showing or satisfying our ego. We should surrender our selfless work to the Divine. It is the best way for purification of Antahkarana. Ego does not involve in this selfless service. We know that every one of us is the embodiment of God. We all are equal. 'Nar seva is the Narayan Sewa'. In other words to reach God serve the mankind.

5. Yoga Nidra:

A yogi enjoys a special type sleep, known as 'chetan Nidra'. It has two benefits. (1). Complete rest (2). Cleanliness of subconscious mind and Antahkarana. It plays an important role removing tension and diseases also. There are some steps given here for help and guidance. Resting in Shavasana mental observation of the body, concentration on breathing, concentration/meditation on five elements, as earth, water, air, fire and aakash Tattva (Ether). Give auto-suggestion for purification/pain in a particular part of the body are quite helpful.

Don't sleep while practising yoga-Nidra. Every point and organ of the body has to be relaxed.

6. Trataka:

It is a part of shatkarma. It is an important kriya for chitta-shuddhi (consciousness purification). It is a steady gazing at a point without blinking. There are two types of trataka 1. External 2. Internal. It improves the eye sight, develops the will power and the concentration of mind. It destroys sanskaras of Chitta. Trataka can be done gazing at moon, candle flame, star, tree, deepak etc. Gazing without winking again and again until the water comes from the eys. Perform palming after that. Wash the eyes with cold water. Avoid its practice in summer.

7. Introspection:

Introspection is a very useful technique before going to bed. Whatever we had decided the last evening try to follow it with a determination. Evaluate properly at night time while sitting for meditation. Inflict self punishment by repenting over the failing or mistakes. For example, suppose we are fond of taking repeated cups of tea, resolve that we will not take tea for a week or so. Besides, take a vow to give-up favourite dish or object or a bad habit.

Sit in padmasana or sukhasana. Whatever work has been done from dawn to dusk, observe it serially and ponder over it. Retrospect whether the duty was performed rightly or wrongly if done wrongly, take a vow not to repeat it the next day. Thus evaluate and remove the mistakes. The consciousness will get purified.

8. Inner Silence (Maun):

Inner Silence means 'Antar Mouna'. In this practice we become aware of the inner world. Though we practice it for a short period each day, this practice extends into our every waking moment and can be practiced for 24 hour a day, anywhere and at any time. It is purely and simply the cultivation of internal awareness of thought, emotional reactions and purification of consciousness.

In the **first stage** we become aware of external sounds and sensations. Don't fight with your mind, don't struggle with the sense experiences but become aware or become a spectator of them. Neither sound, sight, taste, touch, smell, nor anything else should disturb you. The senses are calmed by the attitude of 'I am the seer of experiences'. Be an observer, a witness of the interaction between sound and the ears. This part can be practiced anywhere and at anytime.

Stage 2 means the withdrawal of awareness from the out-side into the mind, the thinking process, the awareness of the spontaneous thoughts that come and go of their own accord. We should remain a silent witness of every thought that is going on in our minds. We will find thoughts coming up, unstimulated, insignificant, in the form of a glimpse, in the twinkling of a eye.

Sometimes there is a mental blockage and no thoughts come, it means that the consciousness is not manifesting itself. The mind goes on thinking, but we don't see it. There is a veil covering the thought. There are some thoughts which we don't wish to register in our mind. We want to escape from them.

Don't oppose any thought, don't hesitate, don't suffer from any sense of guilt. Free thinking but vigilant seeing. You are not the thought, but you are the witness of the thought. Absolute detachment. Don't hate any thought, don't like any thought, but allow them to manifest.

Now bring the mind back to the physical body because the Antar mouna is over. Recite Aum sound loudly.

Note:

1. **Control over one's tongue:** Speak what is necessary.
2. **Control speech:** Don't utter a word and maintain absolute calmness.
3. **Inner silence:** Observe the thoughts with the mind's eye when sushumna nadi gets activated.

9. Prayer:

Prayer means heartily aspiration. The true prayer is that sweet impulse that rises in one's heart for being granted naturally and spontaneously. Never does sincere (truthful) prayer go unanswered. The prayer is a simple and yet a miraculous technique in which we feel God nearby. All our sins are pardoned. Prayer purifies our consciousness. The faults of attachment, hatred, fear, anger and Jealousy etc, melt away. Vedic prayers are very effective. You can make your own prayer according to your situation.

10. Sattvic Diet:

That diet which augments the balanced state of body and mind is said to be sattvic diet. In India this diet consists of fruit, nuts, milk/milk products, steamed vegetables, cooked grains, beans and lentils. These foods are said to increase sattva in the body because they are light, simple and supply all the essential nutrients. At the same time they increase our mental and physical vitality so that we can move easily, experience peace, bliss, lightness and clarity of mind. Sattvic food is the cause of our sattvic thoughts.

- Avoid Rajsic and Tamsic food as narrated in Geeta.
- Take food only when you feel hungry.
- While taking meals fill half of the stomach with food. Leave $1/4^{th}$ part of it for air and the remaining $1/4^{th}$ for water.

- Chew the articles of food properly and take water in small draughts (at least an hour after meals).
- Surrender first to Divine the food doing prayer and eat it in calmful state.
- Eat the food when the air blows from the right-nostril. Drink the water when the air blows from the left nostril.
- Weekly fast recommended living on water, lemon, honey or orange etc.

• • •

16

Yoga and Sex

Sex is neither good nor bad, wrong nor sinful. It depends on the way. We regard sex. Sex is necessary for the procreation of the species and as an act of love. It is uplifting and of immense benefit to health and happiness. As an instrument of lust, however, it degrades and when uncontrolled makes man a slave, leads to dishonesty, deceit, vulgarity and meanness. It is human to err and sensuality can be rectified by developing character. For without character one can't truly love. By yogic techniques it is possible to distinguish between love and lust, and thus not delude ourselves. The present permissive society is not so antithesis of yoga.

Sex and Emotions

Sex is disproportionate with regard to the emotions. Emotions affect breathing, blood circulation, glands, organs, skin, eyes, ears, touch and taste, all of which are conditioned by the right or wrong use of sex. As a result health can be improved or destroyed. Rules, regulations and knowledge about sex and its functions are laid down in the kaam sutras, which are not pornographic but educative.

Role of Yoga

If we do not control, or feel at home with the sexual urge/ feeling, we invite mental and physical diseases. Celibacy is the best way to control the energy. Marriage is the means of utilisation of physical/sexual energy but in a limit. It helps to balance the sex.

Yoga invented many echniques to control and sublimate the sexual energy which is helpful for sound health, mental power and to awaken the kundalini or achieve the state of realisation. Yoga can help to control on this instinct which can otherwise leads us to animal like behaviour.

Sexual energy is life energy. If we save it, sublimate it, we can make our nerves, mind and 'will power' strong. We can also transform this energy into Divine Bliss (Ananda) Divine light, Creative force and longevity. Our sex organs glands become healthy and calm.

Asanas, Pranayama, Mudras, meditation, yama, niyama are the tools for sexual discipline and celibacy. The liberation of the spirit comes through release of the sexual impulse. Failing of vitality in middle age, sex disability can be cured by proper diet, adequate rest, cultivation of relaxed attitude and yogabhyasa.

Developing the Sexual Energy

There are many techniques designed for this purpose such as–sheersasana, Sarvangasana or half sarvangasana, paschimottansana, garudasana, halasana, matsyasana, ardhamatsyendrasana, ashvini mudra, vajroli, uddiyanabandha, pranayama (solar plexus breath) meditation, shavasana etc.

Menopause Situation

When a woman crosses the age of forty she has to face the terrible situation–menopause. Yoga gives her a confidence and help. Triangle (Trikon) asana, rocking exercise (Dolanasana). Sarvangasana, Sheersasana, cobra pose, shavasana, Nauli kriya and uddiyanbandha help a lot. Avoid taking stimulating food and drink. Take plenty of rest, fresh air. Be busy in a work or hobby. Calmness, balanced mind, etc. Remove depression, sense of rejection, selfpity, gloomy thoughts and lack of confidence.

Control of Sexual feelings (Kaam Vasana)

If you are feeling the sexual feelings or irritation you should bring awareness, Relax your body by shavasana. Perform pranayama-kapalbhati, deep breathing, sheetali; Paschimottanasana, utkatasan, padangusthasana, matsyasana, paryankasana, ardhasarvangasana. Vipreet Karani mudra and shavasana. Don't accept the sexual urge. Try to save your energy. Call for the Divine help. Your prayer will be answered.

Sublimation of Energy

Very few people know about the energy in the physical body. There are five energies such as: (1) Mental energy (2) Physical energy (3) Sexual energy. These can be interchanged (4) Energy of intellect and (5) Energy of the soul.

These are independent and indestructible. Physical energy may be transformed into mental/sexual energy. Sexual energy may be transformed into physical or mental energy by Kundalini Yoga.

Kundalini or latent nervous power, is described as a "coiled serpent sleeping at the base of the spine", and when she is waken by the appropriate practices of mantra, mudra, pranayama, "she uncoils and rushes, hissing up through the spine to the top of the head in Sahasrar.

On her journey from her sleeping place, she passes through the six chakras of the body arousing each one in turn with each chakra "in vibration" the yogi experiences the awakening of different psychic powers associated with them.

Kundalini Yoga demand, such intense accumulation of mental powers that every other possible form of energy must be drawn from the body to strengthen mind. Sexual energy is transmuted into mental energy.

Transmuting Sexual Energy

Method: Sit with thighs crossed so that they over lap each other, with the right foot by the left side of the body and the left foot by the right side. The hands, with fingers stretched, and palms down are placed one upon the other, on the upper knee. Hold the pose, inhaling and exhaling deeply, with the mind concentrated on transmiting sexual energy to the solar plexus. Where it is stored as increased physical energy. It is transmuted to physical level.

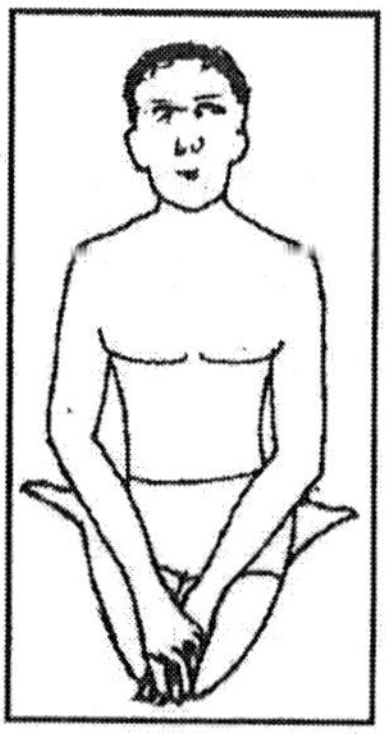

Fig. 134

Note: To transmute the sexual energy to mind energy Sheersasana/Sarvangasana is performed. After the pose breath are established. Imagine that with each incoming breath you are drawing sex energy from the moon Region (Near solar plexus towards and left side) directing it, with each out going breath, up through the spine to the head, where it manifests as increased power of the mind. This is also done in crossed legged pose using same principle.

• • •

17

Yogic Diet

What is Yogic Diet?

Food is an integral part of yoga. It is assumed that vegetarianism is an integral part of yogic practice, because it is light and easy to digest, promotes inner calmness and harmony between the body and mind. Vegetarianism is the basis of a sattvic diet which increases vitality, purity of mind and life span. Yogic diet can be summed up as the most natural and simplest to purchase, to prepare to consume and digest.

"As is the food so is the mind and as the mind so becomes the man." "Right food is the greatest single factor for the promotion of health." "Food is thy medicine and medicine is thy food" "Quality and quantity of food play an important role in the well-being of a person and need consideration." "We eat to live but not live to eat." Yogic diet is an important means of purification, preparing the sadhaka for progress in meditation, yogic sleep and controlling the sexual feelings.

"Yoga is not possible for him who eats too much, nor for him who does not eat at all nor for him who sleeps too much, nor for him who is always awake O!Arjun." Gita Chapter 6/16

The food which increase life, purity, strength, health, joy and cheerfulness (good appetite), which are savoury and oleaginous, substantial and agreeable are dear to the sattvic (Pure). Gita Chapter. 17/8.

The food that are bitter, sour, saline, excessively hot or cold, pungent, dry and burning are liked by the Rajsic and are productive of pain, grief and disease. Gita Chapter 17/9.

"That which is stale, tasteless, putrid rotten, and impure, is the food liked by the tamsic." Gita Chapter 17/10.

Yogashastra gives much importance to the goodness (Sattvic) of food. Sattvic food consists of fruits, fresh and green vegetables, cereals—Rice, Barley, Wheat, Cow milk, Curd, Buttermilk, Butter, Ghee, Mash, Sugar (Jaggery), Sugarcandy, Honey, Jujube, Dried ginger, Jack fruit, Nut, Salad, of Carrot, Radish, Cucumber, cauliflower; Khichri (combination of rice & Lentils. Vegetables, salt according taste and one spoon turmeric) sprouted cereals, Soyabeans, basil, lemon amla dry fruits etc.

Needs of the Body

The first step is to understand basic food values and learn what constitutes a balance diet. Dieticians, doctors and scientists tell us that our food must contain health-giving constituents. If our bodies are to function properly. The health-giving constituents are listed below:

S.N.	Components	Purpose	Sources
1.	Protein	Growth and the repair of body tissue to satisfy the hunger	Dairy products, soyabeans, root vegetables, nuts, pulses, wholegrain cereals, whole meal flour and bread gram, ground nut, peas.
2.	Vitamins Vitamin A	Helps to build and mend body tissues for fighting disease	Dairy products (milk, butter and cheese) leafy and green vegetables, carrot watercress, tomato, prunes, figs, oranges, dry fruits.

	Vitamin B	For healthy muscular and nervous system utilisation of carbo -hydrates.	Whole meal bread and flour, peanuts lentils, leafy and green vegetables, soya beans yeast, dairy products, yogurt, oatmeal, sprouted pulses, apple.
	Vitamin C	For vitality/building and mending body tissues	Citrus fruits, fresh fruits, tomato, potato, jackets, lemon, amla, spinach, leafy and green vegetables, peppers cauliflower and water cress, orange.
	Vitamin D	For healthy teeth and bones	Sun rays,: milk, ghee, butter.
3.	**Carbohydrates** (starchy, sugary food)	Provide heat and energy, for assimilation action and digestion to build muscles, stimulating the large intestines to help prevent constipation.	Grains, pulses, rice, potato dry fruits, dates sugar, honey, milk, green leafy and root vegetables, mango, grapes, flour, sugarcane, beans.
4.	**Fat**	Energy and warmth protection from injury or jolts, proper working order of the organs to keep the body stout and beautiful.	Butter, curd, ghee, oil, milk, ground nut, coconut dry-fruits, vegetables oils etc.
5.	**Minerals (salts)** calcium, phosphorus, iron, sodium chloride, potassium, iodine, magnesium chlorine, copper, sulphur, flourine, manganese, water.	Functioing of different body systems bone and body growth, maintaining acid equilibrium generating blood, harmone formation generating stomach juices, thyroxin and teeth enamel etc.	Green and leafy vegetables fruits and dry fruits, (apple, pineapple, grapes banana, mango) sprouted pulses, ground nuts, dates, sea salt, garlic, water nut, milk and milk products, soyabean, coco nut, juggery wal nut, pudina, methi, chaulai, lemon, cereal, pulses, resin, grams, beetroot etc.

Useful Hints about Food

1. **Selectivity:** Choose only pure food to reduce all possible inner pollution. Diet is a very individual affair. Peoples requirements vary according to the work they do and the amount of energy they need. Everyone should study his own personal needs and biological type so that by the time he reaches middle age he has a good idea of what foods suit him the best.
2. **Moderation:** It is the second step. Eat which is tasty, at the proper time, suitable and beneficial to health and fully controlled.
   - One should fill half the stomach with solid food and leave one fourth for water and one fourth for air.
   - You should eat only when you feel hungry.
   - Keep meals simple, not eating too many different foods all together because this habit disturbs the metabolic balance.
   - Don't be influenced by fashions, friends or magazine or news paper's "new idea".
   - Eat less and live longer. Excess in eating causes diabetes, gout, blood pressure, heart disease, dyspepsia, piles and other ailments.
3. **Mastication:** It is third important rule. Chew every thing thoroughly and remember that digestion begins in the mouth.
   - Mastication every morsel of food to such extent that it becomes liquid and automatically goes down your throat.
   - With mastication you can save yourself from overeating.
   - While you masticate the morsel think in your mind. "I am drawing 'pran' from every morsel my body is being strong."
   - Avoid talking at the time of mastication and keep away feelings of doubts, fear, anger, stress, irritation. Eat with happy mood and peaceful attitude. Concentrate on food

and feel, "**My digesting power is increasing. I am feeling hunger. My stomach is strong. The digesting process in working smoothly. The blood is being pure. I am eating powerful, peaceful and satisfying food.**"

4. **Prayer:** Select a clean place. Sit on an aasan. Be silent. Pray to God before eating and thank Him for his kindness after eating.
5. Never eat anything either **too hot** or **cold**. Ice cold food and beverage have an injurious effect on teeth, tongue, stomach and gallbladder. Too hot foods destroy the teeth.
6. **Water:** Never drink water during meals. If done otherwise the digestive juices are diluted and obstruct and impede the process of digestion. Drink water one hour before or one hour after the meals.
7. **Combination of Foods:** It is very very important. Fruits should always be taken as a separate meal and never in combination with vegetables and starchy foods. It is better to eat a monodiet.
   - The general rule to be followed is that the easily digestive ones to follow the ones harder to digest also solids the follow liquids.
8. **Posture:** The ideal posture while eating is the squating/crossed legged on the floor. The trunk should be slightly bent forward while taking the morsel in.
   - Sit in Vajrasana after the meals. After meals lie down on left side. Walking is beneficial after dinner and it is good for digestion.
9. Avoid strenuous work immediately after meals Cycling, performing yogasana, swimming, sexual intercourse are harmful just after the meals.
10. **Fasting:** If you are not hungry, don't eat. Miss a meal; miss two meals, miss a whole day of meals and you will feel all the more better for it. Drink lemon and honey water or

honey and water or juice several times. If needed take enema. Bowls will be cleared.

Weekly fasting is good but 2-3 days fast with in a month is very beneficial. Mind it never take heavy and solid food just after the fast. Senior citizens should avoid their dinner and they should take light food or fruits, mash or milk.

11. **Injurious foods:** Excessive salt, chilly and spices, fried and roasted spicy vegetables, vanaspati ghee, sweatmeats, vinegar, skinned pulses, poori, biscuits, ice-cream, tea-coffee, white sugar, polished rice, soft drinks, tinned milk and meals, alcohol, tobacco, egg, meat, fish, maida, finely grounded and stale flour, unseasonal fruits etc. are avoidable food stuffs as they execute the digestive system against its nature.
12. **Cleanliness:** Cleanliness is next to God. It has an important place in food. Utenscils, place and hands should be neat and clean. Wash hands before eating any thing. Wash properly vegetables and fruits before use.
13. **Never eat many times:** Not a single morsel of food should be eaten between any two meals because the digestive juices go waste if we just eat something in between the meals.
14. Eat your evening meal at least two to there hours before going to bed. Late dinners are positively harmful and must be avoided. There should be four to six hours gap between two meals.
15. Don't take the next meal until the first meal has been digested.
16. Take only fresh meal, stored foods for a long time are harmful. Don't eat chopped, dust-exposed or fly ridden food.
17. Eat salad, chapati/rice and pulse, curd/buttermilk at lunch or dinner. Soup daliya fruit, milk, lemon, honey mixed in luke warm water at break fast and tiffin time.
18. Know the food value you take in.

• • •

Other Books on

HEALTH BOOKS

1. Child Development (New)
2. Yoga for Health and Relaxation
3. Yoga For Daily Life (New)
4. A Guide to Your Pregnancy (New)
5. Ayurveda for All (New)
6. A Guide to Migraine, Airthritis, Cervical Spondylosis, and Backache (New)
7. Body and Beauty Care (New)
8. Yoga for All (New)
9. Child Care and Nutrition
10. Naturopathy Modern Way of Life
11. First Aid How to Handle an Accident
12. Acupressure in Daily Life
13. Complete Book of Yoga
14. Look Younger at Any Age
15. HIV/AIDS - Transmission, Prevention & Alternative Therapies
16. Diabetics and Diet
17. Increase your Height & Loose your Weight
18. Make Fitness A Way of Life
19. Common Problems of Children
20. Handbook of Nutrition & Dietetics
21. A Guide to Massage Therapy
22. A Guide to Family Medicine
23. A Guide to Digestive Disorders
24. Complete Book of Child Care

25. A Guide to Homoeopathy
26. Life Begins at 40
27. Alternative Therapies
28. How to Overcome Stress
29. Yoga Therapy
30. Obesity
31. Self Motivation
32. Women Disorders and Pregnancy
33. A Guide to Body Pains
34. Sex Education
35. Common Diseases and Cure
36. Pranayama for Better Life
37. Herbal Home Remedies
38. A Guide to Beauty & Skin Care
39. A Guide to Heart Care
40. A Guide to High Blood Pressure
41. Cancer Causes and Prevention
42. Nature Cure for Common Diseases
43. Good Health Through Food and Regimen
44. A Guide to Allergies
45. A Guide to Aging
46. Ayurveda for Health & Beauty

Lotus PRESS